Working in Health

Working in Health

Financing and Managing the Public Sector Health Workforce

Marko Vujicic
Kelechi Ohiri
Susan Sparkes

With contributions from
Aly Sy
Tim Martineau
Christoph Kurowski
Claudia Rozas
Andrew Mitchell
Kyla Hayford
and Sherry Madan

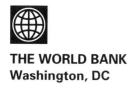

THE WORLD BANK
Washington, DC

1818 H Street NW
Washington DC 20433
Telephone: 202-473-1000
Internet: www.worldbank.org
E-mail: feedback@worldbank.org

ISBN-13: 978-0-8213-7802-1
eISBN: 978-0-8213-7803-8
DOI: 10.1596/978-0-8213-7802-1

Library of Congress Cataloging-in-Publication Data

Vujicic, Marko.
Working in health : financing and managing the public sector health workforce / Marko Vujicic, Kelechi Ohiri, and Susan Sparkes ; with Tim Martineau ... [et al.].
    p. ; cm. — (Directions in development)
    Includes bibliographical references and index.
    ISBN 978-0-8213-7802-1 (alk. paper)
    1. Public health personnel—Salaries, etc.—Developing countries. 2. Medical economics—Developing countries. I. Ohiri, Kelechi. II. Sparkes, Susan. III. World Bank. IV. Title. V. Series: Directions in development (Washington, D.C.)
    [DNLM: 1. Health Manpower—economics—Dominican Republic. 2. Health Manpower—economics—Kenya. 3. Health Manpower—economics—Rwanda. 4. Health Manpower—economics—Zambia. 5. Health Manpower—organization & administration—Dominican Republic. 6. Health Manpower—organization & administration—Kenya. 7. Health Manpower—organization & administration—Rwanda. 8. Health Manpower—organization & administration—Zambia. 9. Developing Countries—Dominican Republic. 10. Developing Countries—Kenya. 11. Developing Countries—Rwanda. 12. Developing Countries—Zambia. 13. Salaries and Fringe Benefits—legislation & jurisprudence—Dominican Republic. 14. Salaries and Fringe Benefits—legislation & jurisprudence—Kenya. 15. Salaries and Fringe Benefits—legislation & jurisprudence—Rwanda. 16. Salaries and Fringe Benefits—legislation & jurisprudence—Zambia. W 76 V989w 2009]
    RA410.55.D48V85 2009
    362.1—dc22

                                                                                    2008051555

Cover image: Photo Courtesy of the Bill & Melinda Gates Foundation
Cover design: Quantum Think

Contents

Boxes

Figures

Tables

Foreword

Health is at the center of the global development agenda, with four of the eight Millennium Development Goals (MDGs) focused on health. The past few years have brought a remarkable increase in donor assistance to developing countries, bringing real opportunities to improve the health of poor people.

At the center of every health system are health workers, but staffing levels in many developing countries—particularly in Sub-Saharan Africa—are far below the levels needed to deliver essential health services. Inequitable geographic distribution, inappropriate skill mix, low productivity, and poor quality of care delivered are important factors that limit the effectiveness of the workforce. Addressing these health workforce challenges is essential to reach the MDGs.

Numerous factors limit the ability to scale up the health workforce in developing countries. They include insufficient training capacity, health workers choosing not to work in health-related occupations, and migration. However, much of the debate has focused on how restrictive government wage bill policies have affected the health workforce. When governments limit the expansion of the overall wage bill—often for sound fiscal policy reasons—this restriction is thought to lead to insufficient resources for hiring new health workers. Despite a critical need, however, little information is available about how fiscal policy affects the health workforce.

Similarly, public sector policies and practices for recruiting, deploying, promoting, and paying health workers are important determinants of geographic distribution, skill mix, and productivity as well as the quality of care provided by the workforce. But these processes also are not well documented.

This book examines two key health workforce policy questions:

- What is the impact of government wage bill policies on the size of the health wage bill and on health workforce staffing levels in the public sector?
- Do current human resource management policies and practices lead to strategic use of health wage bill resources in the public sector?

Through country case studies in Kenya, Zambia, Rwanda, and the Dominican Republic, this book demonstrates that an analysis of wage bill budget trends, budget execution rates, vacancies, and unemployment levels among health workers can be used to determine whether fiscal ceilings are preventing scaling up the health workforce. Such a methodology was not previously available and is a useful tool for policy makers. The book also reviews the literature and analyzes available administrative data on a broader sample of countries.

The analysis found that wage bill restrictions were a significant constraint to scaling up the health workforce in only one of the four countries studied in depth. However, in all four cases, significant weaknesses were found in policies and practices related to recruitment, deployment, transfer, promotion, sanctioning, and payment methods of public sector health workers. Recruitment processes are plagued by delays and not targeted to areas with staff shortages. Salaries and allowances are not being used to provide strong incentives for increasing rural practice and lowering absenteeism. Available wage bill resources are often not fully spent, and even when they are, considerable scope is available to use these resources more strategically. Thus, improving recruitment, deployment, transfer, promotion, and remuneration practices is just as important—and maybe more important—than expanding the health wage bill in addressing health workforce challenges.

The health workforce challenges in developing countries are significant, but the evidence base for policy makers is weak. This book is an important initial contribution to the evidence base in fiscal policy and public sector management. The World Bank will continue its commitment to this unfinished agenda.

Julian Schweitzer
Director
Health, Nutrition, and Population
The World Bank

Acknowledgments

This report was prepared by a core team consisting of Marko Vujicic (task team leader); Kelechi Ohiri (McKinsey & Company, formerly World Bank); and Susan Sparkes through generous funding support from the Bill & Melinda Gates Foundation and the Ministry of Foreign Affairs, Government of Norway.

Several others contributed to the report. Tim Martineau (Liverpool Associates in Tropical Health) completed the initial fieldwork and early drafts of case studies for Kenya and Zambia. Consultants Aly Sy and Claudia Rozas carried out the initial fieldwork and prepared early drafts of case studies for Rwanda and the Dominican Republic, respectively. Consultant Chresta Kaluba worked with the core team in Zambia to complete the case study. Consultants Andrew Mitchell, Kyla Hayford, and Sherry Madan carried out the analysis and coauthored appendixes C, D, and E, respectively, with the core team. Consultants Chai Hapugalle and Vandana Ashton assisted in editing the report. Inputs were also received from Valerie Moran.

Throughout the writing of this report, the core team benefited from insightful comments and guidance of Christoph Kurowski, who also helped oversee the Dominican Republic case study, and Ajay Tandon. The team is grateful for feedback from peer reviewers Keith Hansen, Timothy

Johnston, and Kees Kostermans. Helpful comments on earlier drafts as well as suggestions for data and information sources were received from Mukesh Chawla, Pablo Gottret, Dominic Haazen, Christopher Herbst, Adam Lagerstedt, Michael Mills, David Peters (Johns Hopkins University), Oscar Picazo, Gary Reid, George Schieber, Agnes Soucat, Rosemary Sunkutu, Marijn Verhoeven, and Monique Vledder.

Executive Summary

The health workforce plays a key role in increasing access to health services for the poor in developing countries. Recent evidence has demonstrated an important link between staffing levels and both service delivery and health outcomes. Various global and country-level estimates have also shown that current staffing levels in developing countries—particularly in Sub-Saharan Africa—are often well below those required to deliver essential health services.

Several factors potentially limit increasing the number of health workers in developing countries. They include insufficient training capacity, health workers choosing not to work in health occupations, low labor force participation rates, and net migration flows. One extremely important factor that has received considerable attention in recent years is restrictive overall wage bill policy within the public sector. A large share of the health workforce in developing countries is employed in the public sector. As a result, health workers' salaries are paid from the government's overall wage bill budget. When governments decide to limit the expansion of the overall wage bill—often for very sound economic reasons—this policy can lead to insufficient resources for hiring health workers. In fact, much of the global debate has focused heavily on this fiscal constraint and how it is *the* key factor that limits scaling up the health workforce. Despite a critical need, however, little empirical evidence is available.

Numbers are not everything. Although the global debate has focused on shortages and the need to increase the number of health workers in developing countries, strong evidence indicates that geographic distribution, skill mix, productivity, and quality of care are just as important in improving service delivery and health outcomes. Within the public sector, government policies and practices related to recruitment, deployment, promotion, sanctioning, and remuneration methods for health workers influence these factors heavily. In these areas, too, very little country experience has been documented.

This report addresses two key policy questions:

- What is the impact of government wage bill policies on the size of the health wage bill and on health workforce staffing levels in the public sector?
- Do current human resource management policies and practices lead to strategic use of health wage bill resources in the public sector?

The relevant literature was examined, and available cross-country data were analyzed. Detailed country-level work was also carried out in four focus countries: Kenya, Zambia, Rwanda, and the Dominican Republic. Governments in all of these countries recently went through periods of scaling back their overall wage bill. Against this backdrop, the health sector strategy in each of the countries clearly identifies a need for additional wage bill resources in the health sector. Thus, the tension between the fiscal constraint on the overall wage bill at the central level and the sector goal to expand the health wage bill is common across these countries. But the policy approach to resolving this tension and the actual effect on budgets and staffing levels are quite different in each country, providing rich lessons learned. Differences in policies and practices for key human resource management functions also occur, both across countries and within countries over time, providing insight on how wage bill resources can be used more effectively.

The Impact of Government Wage Bill Policies on the Health Wage Bill and Hiring of Health Workers

Under the first policy question, the report examines how overall government wage bill policies affect the size of the health wage bill, the ability to scale up hiring of health workers in the public sector, and the related policy options.

To answer the first policy question, the case studies reviewed the budgeting process for the health wage bill in the public sector. This review allowed a better understanding of the actors involved and the processes through which fiscal policies influence the health wage bill. Trends in the overall public sector wage bill, the budget for the health wage bill (including how vacancies are created), and budget execution rates (that is, whether budgeted money was actually spent) were analyzed. This information was compared with hiring trends and staffing levels for health workers in the public sector.

The key findings follow:

- A strong economic rationale exists for controlling the size of the overall public sector wage bill. Countries implement restrictive overall wage bill policies for a variety of reasons, but they are usually only a short-term policy response.
- Wage bill ceilings are a common conditionality of International Monetary Fund (IMF) lending, but the IMF has recently concluded that wage bill ceilings have been overused within its programs. When the health wage bill is part of the government's overall wage bill, the ministry of health has relatively little control over the size of its health wage bill budget.
- The wage bill budgeting process provides scope for governments to prioritize the health sector over other sectors. However, the stated government policy of prioritizing the health sector within the overall wage bill does not always translate into practice.
- Increasing the health wage bill—even significantly—need not lead to unsustainable growth in the overall wage bill. However, when wage increases or expanded hiring spill over into other sectors, the fiscal impact on the overall wage bill can be considerable.
- Government overall wage bill policies can have important implications for the health workforce. However, the effect is by no means consistent across countries. In only one of the four country case studies did evidence show that wage bill restrictions were a significant constraint to scaling up the health workforce.
- A careful analysis of wage bill budget levels, wage bill budget execution rates, vacancies, hiring trends, and unemployment among health workers needs to be carried out to determine whether restrictions on the overall wage bill are an important constraint to scaling up the health workforce. This analysis must be done on a country-by-country basis.

Human Resources Management Policies and Practices and Their Effect on Strategic Use of Wage Bill Resources

Under the second policy question, the report examines how well health wage bill resources are used in the public sector. The case studies reviewed the policies and practices related to key human resource management functions within the public sector in the four focus countries. The functions examined included recruitment, deployment, transfer, promotion, and sanctioning of health workers. Policies and practices related to the types of contracts and methods of remuneration and other incentives were also reviewed. Policies and practices related to these functions were then linked to selected outcomes, including budget execution rate for the health wage bill, geographic distribution, and absenteeism of staff members.

The key findings follow:

• The recruitment process is often plagued by considerable delays and is not targeted to areas with the highest need for staff.
• Formal legislation governs termination and sanctioning of civil service employees, but the formal policy can be very different from the actual practice.
• More strategic management of promotions and transfers can improve the geographic distribution of workers.
• Salaries are often not linked to posts. Linking salaries to posts rather than to people is an effective method of addressing geographic inequities in staffing.
• Allowances are an important part of remuneration for individual health workers and account for a significant part of the health wage bill, but they are often not used strategically.
• Overall, in all four country case studies, significant weaknesses were found in policies and practices related to recruitment, deployment, transfer, promotion, sanctioning, and payment methods of health workers in the public sector. These weaknesses contribute to low budget execution rates for the health wage bill, geographic inequities in staffing levels, and absenteeism. Considerable scope exists to use current health wage bill resources much more strategically.

Policy Options to Address Fiscal Constraints on the Health Wage Bill and to Improve Management of the Health Workforce in the Public Sector

Governments might consider several policy options to address the fiscal constraints to expanding the health wage bill (where they arise) and to improve key human resource management policies and practices that affect how health wage bill resources are used. These policy options are not intended as prescriptive recommendations, nor is the evidence supporting each policy option fully summarized in this report. Rather, the challenges and the enabling and inhibiting factors for success associated with each policy option are discussed at length to identify where each policy option may be most appropriate. Some of these policy options require significant public sector reform, with considerable risk. Others are more conservative and can be implemented very rapidly within the existing administrative environment.

The policy options include the following:

- Lines of accountability could be strengthened, the information base could be improved, and capacity within the ministry of health could be strengthened to bring current human resource management practices more in line with stated policies.
- Where the ministry of health has autonomy, allowances could be used much more strategically, and alternatives to salary payment could be considered to strengthen the incentives for good performance.
- Within the current budgeting process, the predictability of the health wage bill could be improved by budgeting for a longer period.
- The position of the ministry of health in wage bill budget negotiations could be strengthened so that an increasing share of the overall wage bill is devoted to the health sector.
- Subject to certain conditions, the fiscal constraint on the overall wage bill could be relaxed to accommodate expansion of the health wage bill.
- By working with international agencies, governments could reduce the volatility and unpredictability of donor assistance. Greater predictability could allow more donor assistance for health to be devoted to remuneration of health workers.
- Subject to certain conditions, authority over selected human resources for health functions could be transferred to the ministry of health, while the health wage bill is retained within the overall wage bill.
- Subject to certain conditions—including adequate human resource management capacity—key human resource management functions could be transferred from the central level to the local level.
- Subject to certain conditions, health workers could be removed from the civil service and the overall wage bill so that the ministry of health has full control over both the size and the use of the health wage bill.

Abbreviations

AIDS	acquired immunodeficiency syndrome
BFP	budget framework paper (Rwanda)
BSP	budget strategy paper (Kenya)
CBOH	Central Board of Health (Zambia)
CEPEX	Central Public Investments and External Finance Bureau (Rwanda)
CSA	civil service and administrative (reform)
DHMT	District Health Management Team (Zambia)
DHR&A	Directorate of Human Resources and Administration (Zambia)
DPM	Department of Personnel Management (Kenya)
DSC	district service commission (Uganda)
EDPRS	Economic Development and Poverty Reduction Strategy (Rwanda)
EHP	Emergency Hiring Program (Kenya)
FFS	fee-for-service (system)
GAVI	Global Alliance for Vaccines and Immunization
GDP	gross domestic product
GFATM	Global Fund to Fight AIDS, Tuberculosis, and Malaria
GSS	General Salary Scale (Zambia)

HIV	human immunodeficiency virus
HRH	human resources for health
HSS	health systems strengthening
IDSS	Istituto de Seguros Sociales (Social Security Institute) (Dominican Republic)
IMF	International Monetary Fund
MDG	Millennium Development Goal
MDS	Medical Doctor Salary Scale (Zambia)
MIFOTRA	Ministry of Public Service and Labour (Rwanda)
MINECOFIN	Ministry of Finance and Economic Planning (Rwanda)
MINEDUC	Ministry of Education (Rwanda)
MINISANTE	Ministry of Health (Rwanda)
MOF	Ministry of Finance (Dominican Republic)
MOH	Ministry of Health (Zambia)
MSS	Medical Salary Scale (Zambia)
MTEF	Medium-Term Expenditure Framework
MWG	Macroeconomic Working Group (Kenya)
NDP	National Development Plan (Zambia)
NGO	nongovernmental organization
NHS	National Health System (Dominican Republic)
NIS	National Insurance Scheme (Dominican Republic)
PBG	performance-based grant (Rwanda)
PEPFAR	President's Emergency Plan for AIDS Relief (United States)
PER	public expenditure review (Kenya)
PMEC	Payroll Management and Establishment Control (system) (Zambia)
PRGF	Poverty Reduction and Growth Facility
PSC	Public Service Commission (Kenya, Zambia)
PSMD	Public Service Management Division (Zambia)
SESPAS	Secretaría de Estado de Salud Pública y Asistencia Social (Secretariat of Public Health and Social Assistance) (Dominican Republic)
TB	tuberculosis
USAID	U.S. Agency for International Development
WHO	World Health Organization
ZHWRS	Zambia Health Worker Retention Scheme

CHAPTER 1

Overview

The health workforce plays a key role in increasing access to health services for the poor in developing countries. Recent evidence has demonstrated an important link between the number of health workers and both service delivery and health outcomes (Anand and Bärnighausen 2004; Joint Learning Initiative 2004; WHO 2006). At the global level, according to the World Health Organization (WHO), 57 countries have critically low levels of health care workers. WHO guidelines on staffing levels required to achieve selected service delivery targets indicate that these 57 countries together require an additional 4.3 million health workers. More in-depth country-level estimates of health workforce needs show significant shortages as well (Kombe and others 2005; Kurowski and others 2007). But numbers are not everything. Strong evidence indicates that geographic distribution (Dussault and Franceschini 2006; Wagstaff and Claeson 2004; WHO 2006); skill mix (Preker and others 2008; WHO 2007); quality of care provided (Das and Gertler 2007; Das and Hammer 2004); and productivity (Chaudhury and Hammer 2004; Ferrinho and others 2004; Kurowski and others 2007; Ruwoldt and Hassett 2007; Vujicic, Addai, and Bosomprah 2006) of the health workforce are just as important to improving service delivery. Given that the public sector is a major provider of health services in many developing countries and one of the major employers of health workers, these issues are particularly relevant in the public sector (table 1.1).

Table 1.1   Share of Health Services Provided in the Public Sector

Type of service	Share of health services provided in the public sector (%)						
	Dominican Republic (2002)	Kenya (2003)	Rwanda (2000)	Zambia (2001)	Latin American average	Sub-Saharan African average	Global average
Treatment of fever in a public facility	75	63	93	82	76	78	72
Medical treatment of acute respiratory infection	77	65	91	85	80	79	72
Medical treatment of diarrhea	77	68	95	83	78	80	72
Delivery in a facility	78	65	91	79	85	86	84

Source: Gwatkin and others 2007.

Numerous factors limit scaling up health workforce capacity in developing countries. Important constraints include insufficient training capacity (Preker and others 2008; WHO 2006); the decision of health workers not to work in health-related occupations (Dussault and Vujicic 2008; Vujicic and Evans 2005); and net migration flows (OECD 2007; WHO 2006). Within the public sector, one extremely important factor that has received considerable attention is the fiscal constraint on the government's overall wage bill (Ambrose 2006; Okuonzi 2004; Ooms and Schrecker 2005). When health workers are employed by the government, they are paid out of the government's overall wage bill budget.[1] Therefore, when governments limit the expansion of the overall wage bill—often for very sound fiscal policy reasons—this limitation can lead to insufficient resources to finance additional hiring of health workers. Restrictive wage bill policies, in turn, are often attributed to the influence of international financial institutions such as the International Monetary Fund (IMF) and the World Bank (Ambrose 2006).

In terms of improving the geographic distribution, skill mix, quality of care provided, and productivity of health workers—health workforce outcomes that relate to how effectively current wage bill resources are used—numerous factors need to be considered. In general, these outcomes are driven by complex interactions among different actors within a highly regulated labor market (Vujicic and Zurn 2006). Within the public sector, these outcomes are also driven by policies and practices related to key human resource management functions, such as recruiting, deploying, promoting, sanctioning, and paying health workers (Franco, Bennett, and Kanfer 2002; Vujicic and Zurn 2006).

This report does not address all the critical health workforce issues previously mentioned, such as training, capacity building, health worker attrition, and migration. Such breadth is beyond the scope of this study. Rather, this report addresses two key policy questions:

- What is the impact of government wage bill policies on the size of the health wage bill and on health workforce staffing levels in the public sector?
- Do current human resource management policies and practices lead to strategic use of health wage bill resources in the public sector?

In addressing these two policy questions, this study focuses on two main aspects of health workforce policy. First, it examines how overall government wage bill policies affect the size of the health wage bill, the hiring of health workers in the public sector, and the related policy options. This focus is important because despite the importance of fiscal constraints on the wage bill—and the persistent debate at the global level—very little documented evidence describes how health wage bill budgets in the public sector are determined, how this action is linked to overall wage bill policies, and how it affects the ability of governments to increase staffing levels in the health sector. Recent work has been mostly limited to examining whether wage bill ceilings in IMF programs restrict the use of donor aid (Fedelino, Schwartz, and Verhoeven 2006; Wood 2006) and how government macroeconomic policies and IMF programs affect health spending (Center for Global Development 2007; Vujicic 2005).

Second, this report looks at how well health wage bill resources are used in the public sector. The report reviews the policies and practices for key human resource management functions for the health workforce in the public sector, how these policies and practices are linked to selected health workforce outcomes, and what the relevant policy options are.

To address the two policy questions, we examined the relevant literature and analyzed available cross-country data. Detailed country-level work was also carried out in four countries: the Dominican Republic, Kenya, Rwanda, and Zambia. To answer the first policy question, we reviewed the budgeting process for the health wage bill in the public sector to better understand the actors involved and the processes through which fiscal policies influence the health wage bill. Trends in the overall public sector wage bill, the budget for the health wage bill (including how vacancies are created), and budget execution rates (that is, whether budgeted money is actually spent) were analyzed. This information was compared to hiring trends and staffing levels for health workers in the public sector.

To answer the second policy question, we reviewed the policies and practices related to key human resource management functions within the public sector. The functions examined include recruitment, deployment, transfer, promotion, and sanctioning of health workers. Policies and practices related to the types of contracts and method of remuneration and other incentives were also reviewed. Policies and practices related to these functions were then linked to selected outcomes, including budget execution rate for the health wage bill, geographic distribution, and productivity of staff.

Figure 1.1 provides a simple illustration of the crucial roles that the wage bill budgeting process and key human resource management functions play in determining health workforce staffing levels and other outcomes.

Figure 1.1   Focus of Report

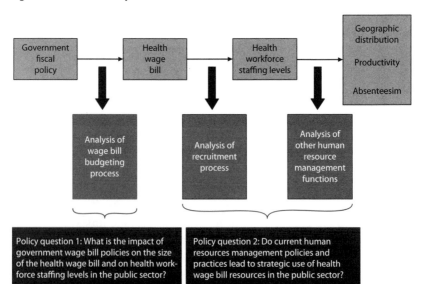

Source: Authors' compilation.

The studied countries were selected on the basis of several factors. Their governments recently went through periods of reduction in the overall wage bill. Against this backdrop, the health sector strategy in each of the countries clearly identifies a need for additional wage bill resources. In Kenya, Rwanda, and Zambia, these resources are mainly needed for substantially scaling up staffing levels to expand health service delivery and meet development priority goals. In the Dominican Republic, additional resources are needed mainly to increase remuneration levels. Thus, the tension between the fiscal constraint on the overall wage bill at the central level and the sector goal to expand the health wage bill is common across the countries. However, the policy approach to resolving this tension and the actual effect on budgets and staffing levels are quite different. Differences in policies and practices for key human resource management functions also exist, both across countries and over time within countries. An examination of these factors provides rich lessons learned related to how strategically wage bill resources are used.

The pattern of health outcomes, service delivery, and health workforce levels in the Dominican Republic, Kenya, Rwanda, and Zambia also suggests that important issues exist with respect to how the health workforce is managed in the public sector. For example, in Kenya, Rwanda, and Zambia, coverage of skilled birth attendance is below average according to several measures, yet overall health worker levels are above average (figure 1.2). This finding suggests that skill mix, geographic distribution, quality of care, or productivity of health workers may be important issues. In the Dominican Republic, health outcomes are below average despite very high health service coverage and high workforce levels, especially for doctors. This finding may suggest a quality of care issue rather than an access issue. A detailed comparative analysis of health outcomes, service delivery, and health workforce levels for the four countries is available in appendix A.

The remainder of this overview chapter is organized as follows. The first section discusses the wage bill budgeting process and is based on the four country case studies, broader cross-country data analysis, and the relevant literature. Primarily using the four country case studies, the second section discusses the effect of the wage bill budgeting process on the health workforce. The third section discusses how wage bill resources are managed in the health sector and is again based primarily on the four country case studies. The fourth section discusses policy options to address the fiscal constraints to scaling up the health workforce and to improve management of wage bill resources. It is based on the four country case studies and the

Figure 1.2   Performance on Selected Health, Service Delivery, and Staffing Outcomes Relative to Income and Health Spending in the Dominican Republic, Kenya, Rwanda, and Zambia, 2005

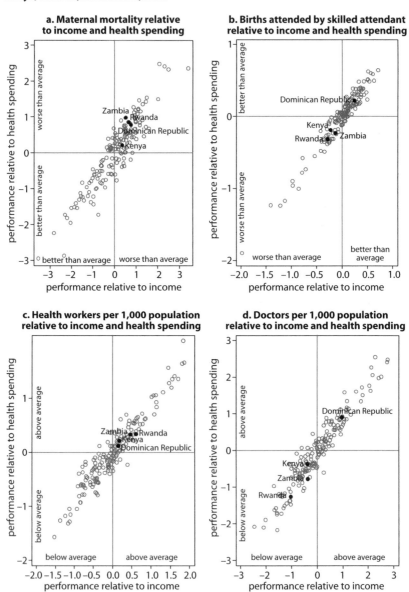

Source: World Bank 2007.

available literature. In this section, the challenges and enabling factors associated with each of the policy options are discussed at length. The discussion makes clear that not all policy options are relevant in many developing countries.

Chapters 2 through 5 provide the country analysis for Kenya, Zambia, Rwanda, and the Dominican Republic, respectively.

Several background analyses referred to throughout chapter 1 are included as appendixes. As noted, appendix A provides a detailed comparative analysis of health outcomes, service delivery, and health workforce levels for the four country case studies. Appendix B provides a summary of stylized facts from a cross-country analysis of health wage bill trends. Appendix C provides a summary of the literature related to decentralization of human resource management functions and how decentralization might improve wage bill management. Appendix D summarizes the literature related to how alternative compensation methods for health workers affect workforce performance. Appendix E analyzes selected issues related to using donor funding for health to finance the health wage bill and the hiring of health workers.

The Wage Bill Budgeting Process in the Public Sector

There is a strong economic rationale for controlling the size of the overall public sector wage bill, but the evidence on what level of spending is too high is not very strong. Individual spending components (including the wage bill) will influence the government's overall contribution to achieving growth and poverty reduction. They can also become important sources of macroeconomic volatility and pressures—for example, when high government wages and large employment push up the wage bill and crowd out other spending, when government wage increases feed into a general wage-price spiral that undermines competitiveness, or when wage increases result in fiscal slippages (Fedelino, Schwartz, and Verhoeven 2006). In practice, whether wage bill spending levels actually lead to macroeconomic instability depends on many factors. For example, where private sector wages follow public sector wages, public wage restraint is particularly important to prevent overall wage inflation. The type of exchange rate regime is also important. Moreover, when wage bill ceilings are implemented, it is usually not because of a thorough analysis of the appropriate share of government spending on wages for the medium term. Rather, it is often a short-term response to an economic crisis. This timing potentially undermines the validity of maintaining such ceilings for lengthy periods. Little evidence addresses what level of spending on the health wage bill is "too high" and triggers the negative effects (Action Aid International 2004; Center for Global Development 2007).

Countries implement restrictive wage bill policies for many reasons, but such policies are usually only short term. In many developing countries, wage bill ceilings usually are put in place when a fiscal crisis occurs or when wage bill expenditures move well beyond what is budgeted—often caused by a breakdown in public sector management (Center for Global Development 2007; Fedelino, Schwartz, and Verhoeven 2006). In other settings, wage bill ceilings may be put in place to help implement broad civil service downsizing policies. Wage bill ceilings usually provide only a short-term fix and ultimately need to be supplanted by civil service reform. Prolonged use of wage bill ceilings may lock in inappropriate civil service structures unless combined with structural reforms to address inefficiencies of civil service employment and pay structures. Often, civil service reform is needed to address problems such as overly compressed wage scales; overstaffing (particularly at lower levels of government); and ineffective promotion, transfer, hiring, and redundancy procedures. In addition, wage ceilings may create incentives to increase nonwage compensation, such as housing allowances and other in-kind benefits. The resulting fragmentation of civil servant remuneration and the proliferation of allowances and benefits obscure the true level of wage-related spending, encourage inequities in compensation, and reduce the overall transparency of such spending (Fedelino, Schwartz, and Verhoeven 2006).

In developing countries that have IMF programs, controlling the size of the overall wage bill is often a focus. Wage bill ceilings are a common conditionality of IMF lending. A recent review found that half of all IMF Poverty Reduction and Growth Facilities (PRGFs) contained some form of wage bill conditionality (Fedelino, Schwartz, and Verhoeven 2006). Conditionality was put in place in countries that had a relatively high wage bill level relative to gross domestic product (GDP) or had government expenditure that was growing at a fast rate. It is recognized that wage bill ceilings need to be accompanied by longer-term civil service reform—they have been used only when first-best solutions have not succeeded and are often used as a last resort. The escalation of wage bill conditionality in Zambia (discussed in chapter 3) is a good example. Moreover, wage bill ceilings within IMF programs never apply to particular sectors but to the overall wage bill only. A review of a sample of

PRGF programs with wage bill conditionally undertaken for this report found only one case (Malawi) where a particular sector, health in this case, was mentioned in the document, and it was mentioned only to explain that additional hiring of health workers had been factored into the wage bill ceiling. As a caveat, even when no specific language indicates which sectors are prioritized, the actual wage bill ceiling levels in IMF programs often take into account the planned hiring or pay increases that will take place in certain sectors. Hiring projections are built into the baseline ceiling (Center for Global Development 2007).

The IMF has recognized that wage bill ceilings have been overused within IMF programs (Verhoeven and Segura 2007). Although wage bill ceilings are useful as a temporary device when a loss of control over payrolls threatens macroeconomic stability, such situations will probably be rare. In practice, they have been used in many other situations—particularly to encourage civil service reform—but often without a clear rationale (Center for Global Development 2007). Critics of wage bill ceilings claim that they have hindered low-income countries from expanding employment in key poverty-reducing areas, such as health and education, and in turn have hurt their ability to achieve the Millennium Development Goals. Recent evidence provides some support for this claim (Center for Global Development 2007). As a result of this criticism and examination of experience, the IMF has reconsidered its position and has issued new guidelines calling for transparent and sufficiently flexible ceilings that can accommodate increased spending in the social sectors—particularly using donor funding. With the strengthening of countries' budgeting and payroll systems, the need for wage bill ceilings will diminish and should be used only in exceptional cases with clear justification, limited duration, sufficient flexibility, and periodic reassessment (Verhoeven and Segura 2007).

The Dominican Republic, Kenya, and Zambia had very restrictive policies governing the overall wage bill and made significant reductions between 2000 and 2008, the period covered by the analysis (figure 1.3). In Rwanda, the overall wage bill has remained fairly stable. For several years, Kenya has had a large public sector wage bill relative to other countries in the region. Since 2003, the size of the overall wage bill has declined significantly to contain a growing budget deficit and to ensure that resources were available for critical nonwage spending. From 2003 to 2006, the IMF included a wage bill ceiling as a condition of lending in the PRGF program. This condition has recently been removed, but the government's most recent budget indicates that cuts to the overall wage bill

[handwritten margin note: Analysis of wage ceilings]

Figure 1.3   Public Sector Wage Bill as a Share of GDP, 2000–08

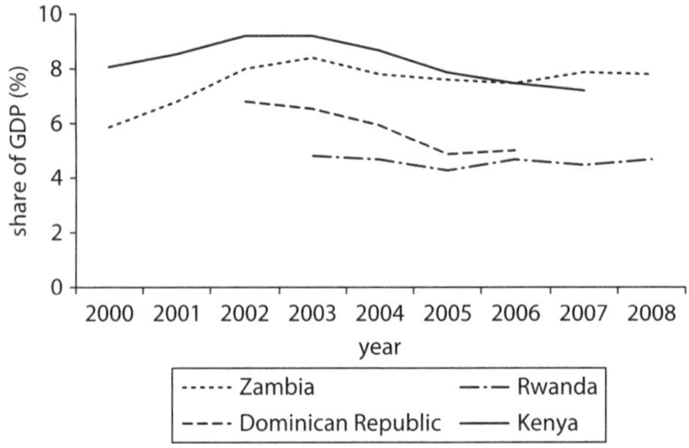

Source: Country case studies.

will continue. In the Dominican Republic, as part of measures taken to resolve the financial crisis in 2002, the government introduced a hiring freeze in the public sector.

From 2000 to 2003, Zambia experienced a sharp increase in the overall public sector wage bill, mainly for reasons other than expanded hiring in priority sectors. During this period, 47 percent of domestic revenue was being used to remunerate civil servants, leaving few resources to finance service delivery and other poverty reduction programs. This trend was deemed unsustainable. To contain the increasing wage bill, the government, in concert with the IMF, made sustainable reductions in public sector wages as a percentage of GDP and brought the public sector wage bill under control.

In 2002, the Dominican economy entered into a recession. The country's public finances were placed under a strain after the government bailed out the country's third-largest bank after a major fraud. The bailout consumed significant government resources and led to an economic crisis. By the end of 2003, inflation reached 42 percent, unemployment stood at 16.5 percent, and the peso had lost more than half its value. As part of the fiscal response, the government implemented significant expenditure controls, including a hiring freeze in the public sector to control the size of the overall wage bill. The hiring freeze remained in effect until 2006.

Although Rwanda has a small overall wage bill compared with that of other countries in the region, the policy priorities of the government of Rwanda are to control spending and to make sure that the wage and salary bill does not get out of control. After cuts in the public workforce brought down the wage bill from 4.8 percent in 2003 to 4.3 percent in 2005, the share of direct wages and salaries in GDP recovered in 2006 to a 4.7 percent level. It is projected to decline briefly in 2007 before remaining stable at 4.7 percent. This reduction shows a concerted effort by the government of Rwanda to reallocate resources away from wages and salaries and toward other budgetary items. Rwanda has never had wage ceilings as a government policy or as a conditionality in PRGFs with the IMF.

In countries where the health wage bill is part of the overall wage bill, the key factor that determines the size of the health wage bill is how governments allocate their overall wage bill budget to different sectors. In all the country case studies, the budgeting process for the health wage bill is similar and generally involves three steps. First, the central authority (for example, the ministry of finance or cabinet) issues budget preparation guidelines instructing line ministries on how to prepare their budgets. *How wage bill gets developed* Sometimes specific instructions related to the wage bill are included in the guidelines. For example, in Kenya in recent years, the budget guidelines have stated that the wage bill for each sector should be set on the basis of current staffing levels, and no increases should be requested. Any incremental resources available for the total public sector wage bill will be allocated to specific sectors only later at the negotiations stage. As part of this first step, line ministries are also required to prepare expenditure reviews that describe what has been accomplished with budget resources from the previous year. Second, a negotiation process takes place in the cabinet, the congress, or the ministry of finance, sometimes involving public hearings, where the central authority debates with line ministries on which sectors should receive additional wage bill resources and which should not. Third, the central authority makes the final decision on the allocation of wage bill resources to different sectors, and this budget is approved by the relevant legal entity. This type of institutional setup has several important implications.

In the four country case studies, the budgeting process for the health wage bill is largely separate from the budgeting process for non-wage health expenditure and is done on a short-term basis. The situation is likely to be the same in countries where the health wage bill is part of the overall wage bill. Essentially, the ministry of health does not have full control over the health wage bill budget. This control ultimately lies with central authorities. The health sector does not receive a certain budget that it then is free to allocate across different inputs to the health care production function. As a result, coordination of the planning of labor and nonlabor inputs within the ministry of health is difficult (figure 1.4). This system may explain why the share of health spending devoted to wages is so volatile over time within countries and varies so widely across countries, as demonstrated in the four case studies and more broadly in appendix B. For example, the share of health spending devoted to wages has fallen considerably in the Dominican Republic despite more of the overall wage bill being devoted to the health sector. Moreover, because budgeting of the health wage bill is often done on a very short-term basis—often for one year only—it is very difficult for ministries of health to plan hiring in the health sector, particularly because health workers are hired mostly on permanent contracts. If wage bill budgets for each sector were planned several years in advance, the ministry of health might more easily plan hiring in the medium to long term. As the institutional arrangement is now, the ministry of health reacts to its wage bill allocation and hires people

Figure 1.4   A Comparison of the Health Wage Bill Budgeting Process

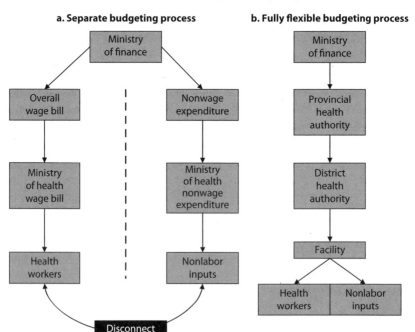

Source: Authors' compilation.

as additional budgets becomes available rather than strategically planning hiring over the medium to long term.

In the four country case studies, the budgeting process provides scope for governments to prioritize certain sectors within the overall wage bill. This is also likely to be the case in other countries where the health wage bill is part of the overall wage bill. The health sector is often singled out as a priority sector for additional hiring within the government's national *HC sector* development plan, as was the case in Kenya, Rwanda, and Zambia. In *thought* Kenya, for example, the government's overall budget strategy documents *of as a* state that, despite the aim to cut the public sector wage bill in Kenya, the *"priority"* health sector remains a priority, and wage bill policy measures will *when* include flexibility to recruit medical personnel. In Zambia, doctors and *making* nurses were specifically excluded from the wage bill freezes that occurred *overall* in 2002 and 2004 in an attempt to prioritize the health sector. In the *wage* Dominican Republic, no explicit policy exempting any sectors from the *bill* hiring freeze was put in place after the economic crisis, but in 2006 doctors and teachers were exempted from a wage freeze that was implemented on all public sector employees.

The key questions, then, are (a) does prioritization of health within the overall wage bill actually occur as the government's policy states, and (b) when it does occur, does it provide enough fiscal space for expanding the health workforce?

The country studies show that the stated policy of prioritizing health within the overall wage bill does not always translate into practice. In the Dominican Republic, Kenya, and Rwanda, the health sector accounted for a steadily increasing share of the overall wage bill, indicating that the health sector was indeed prioritized (figure 1.5). In both Kenya and Rwanda, the government had an explicit policy to prioritize health, but in the Dominican Republic no such policy existed. In Zambia, the share of the overall wage bill going to the health sector decreased steadily during the period of overall wage bill reductions, thus indicating that the wage bill budget of the health sector was cut much more than those of other sectors. In fact, health was not prioritized, in contrast with stated policy; however, the Zambia case is complicated. During the period in question, Zambia was attempting to delink the health sector from the national civil service. When overall wage bill cuts occurred, health workers were being removed from the central payroll and were being hired by local boards of health and paid out of block grants. Whether the delinking process led to a net increase or decrease in the health wage bill as a share of the overall wage bill, however, cannot be ascertained. Accounting

Figure 1.5   Health Wage Bill as a Share of Overall Wage Bill, 2000–07

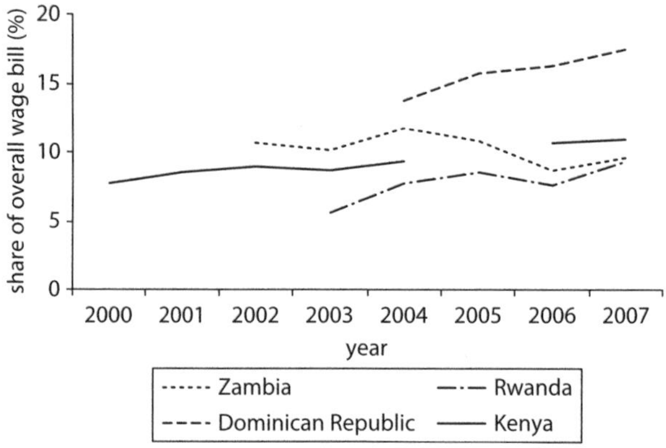

Source: Country case studies.

and data systems used at the time make such an analysis impossible. A further complication is that in 2006 the health sector was relinked, and all staff members are currently in the process of being brought back into the civil service. This series of events could explain the increase in the share of the overall wage bill going to the health sector in recent years, but again, it is impossible to know what share of staff has actually been relinked and what share is still employed by local boards.

Beyond the four country case studies, cross-country data show no clear trend in whether governments are prioritizing the health sector within the overall wage bill. Figure 1.6 plots the percentage change in the overall wage bill against the percentage change in the health wage bill from 2000 to 2004 (latest available aggregate data) in low-income countries. Clearly, some countries shield the health sector when cutting the overall wage bill or prioritize the health sector when the wage bill expands, whereas others target the health sector in times of cuts or prioritize sectors other than health in times of overall wage bill growth. The countries that are above the line are those that prioritized the health sector when cutting or expanding the overall wage bill (that is, the health wage bill is less elastic than the overall wage bill in those countries). The countries below the line are those where the health wage bill expanded more slowly than the overall public sector wage bill, or the health sector wage bill was cut more quickly than the overall wage bill.

Some of the countries plotted in figure 1.6 may have quite different institutional arrangements for employing health workers, which makes

Figure 1.6   Change in Public Sector Health Wage Bill versus Change in Total Public Sector Wage Bill: Sample Countries over Selected Years

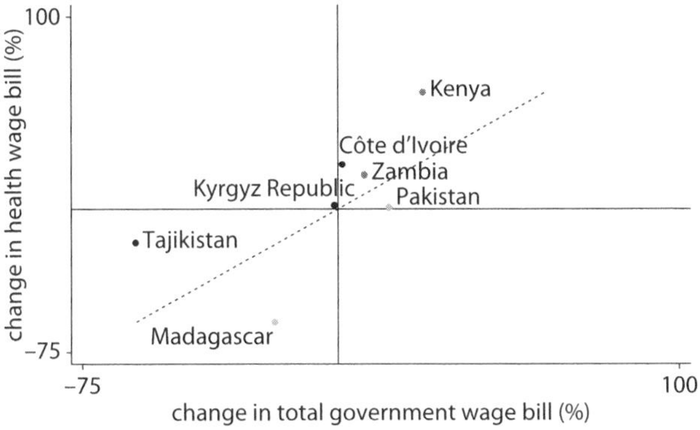

Source: Authors' calculations based on World Bank data.

Note: Côte d'Ivoire, the Kyrgyz Republic, and Tajikistan have prioritized health within the overall government wage bill.

comparisons difficult. For example, in some countries, only a portion of the health wage bill may be included in the overall wage bill (for example, countries where social health insurance is prominent). Because in low-income countries health workers are employed primarily as civil servants (Hongoro and Normand 2006) and social health insurance is not widespread (Gottret and Schieber 2006), only low-income countries were plotted.

Two important observations follow from figure 1.6. First, more countries are above the 45-degree line than below it, indicating general prioritization of the health wage bill within the overall wage in the sample of countries. Second, the slope of the fitted line (not shown) is slightly less than 1, indicating lower volatility of the health wage bill compared with that of the overall wage bill.[2] Of course, because the sample of countries is so small, these conclusions are not reliable.

The country studies have revealed several explanations for why the health sector is not always prioritized in the wage bill allocation decision. In the four country case studies, the degree of transparency in the wage bill budgeting process varies. This factor appears to be important in deciding whether the health sector is prioritized within the process. In Kenya, budget documents are made available to the public at each stage of the process; public hearings are held to get input from the public at large and in general. A Medium-Term Expenditure Framework (MTEF) process is well established in Kenya, and expenditures are monitored to ensure that they are in line with those budgeted in the MTEF. In Zambia, the budgeting process is less transparent. Zambia did not institute an MTEF process until 2003. Even today, the overall wage bill ceiling is adhered to, but allocations of wage bill resources across different ministries often differ from those outlined in the MTEF. For example, the 2007 to 2009 MTEF stated that additional health workers were to be hired over the medium term, but in fact, the initial budgetary allocation from the Ministry of Finance for the health wage bill in 2007 was less than that in 2006. This hypothesis, however, is not supported more broadly in the cross-country analysis. No significant differences occur in the quality of budgeting and financial management levels (as measured by Country Policy and Institutional Assessment scores) between the countries that prioritized the health sector within the overall wage bill and those that did not.

A review of human resources for health (HRH) strategies in 12 countries shows that countries often lack the minimal information set required for strategic planning. HRH strategies tend to focus on estimating staffing needs to achieve ambitious service delivery targets that are often feasible only in the long term. In contrast, when ministries of health present incremental, short-term strategies that are costed with clear priorities and clear, expected health benefits, their negotiating position is strengthened.

In the end, the wage bill allocation decision is a political decision. Different sectors compete against each other for additional wage bill resources. Therefore, it is important for the ministry of health to show how incremental resources will be used and how they benefit the population. The view is often expressed that the health sector is a poor investment of wage bill resources because money is not well spent and because showing how additional resources in previous years were used is difficult (Center for Global Development 2007).[3] Even more fundamentally, often little information is available on how many health workers are employed and where the most crucial shortages are. A review of a sample of HRH strategies in developing countries shows that fewer than half provide costed policy scenarios (table 1.2).

Weak HRH strategies and the nature of the wage bill budgeting process lead the health sector to a low-level equilibrium in terms of the wage bill allocation. Given that the ministry of health does not control the health wage bill and does not know the wage bill envelope for the sector for more than one to three years into the future, strategic planning of human resources for health is difficult to do. Consequently, weak

[handwritten margin note: Implication of HC sector's "low level equilib" allocation level... vicious cycle (cont on next pg)]

Table 1.2   Analysis of National Human Resources for Health Strategies

Country	Overall vision and objectives	Quantifiable targets for staffing	Situational analysis	Short-term projections of staffing levels	Alternative policy scenarios	Clear prioritization and sequencing of actions	Costing of scenarios	Effect of policies on staffing and service delivery
Afghanistan	✓				✓			
Eritrea	✓	✓	✓		✓			✓
Kenya	✓		✓		✓	✓		✓
Lesotho	✓		✓	✓	✓	✓		
Mozambique	✓	✓	✓	✓	✓	✓		✓
Philippines	✓		✓	✓	✓		✓	
Rwanda	✓		✓	✓	✓		✓	✓
Sierra Leone	✓	✓	✓	✓	✓	✓	✓	✓
South Africa	✓		✓	✓	✓	✓		✓
Sudan	✓		✓			✓		
Thailand	✓			✓	✓	✓		✓
Zambia	✓			✓			✓	✓

Source: World Bank staff analysis of national human resources for health strategies.

human resources for health strategies undermine the ministry of health's position in wage bill budget negotiations, thus resulting in little increase in wage bill resources for the health sector. In turn, when the health sector receives fewer wage bill resources, little incentive exists for strategic planning of hiring because budgets are falling.

Prioritizing the health sector in terms of the wage bill budget is sometimes politically difficult. Within a fixed overall wage bill envelope, prioritizing the health wage bill would require reallocating resources away from other sectors. Even if a strong economic or development rationale exists to do so, this course is often politically difficult. Nevertheless, governments in the Dominican Republic, Kenya, and Rwanda and have done it. In the Dominican Republic, prioritization of health and education within the shrinking overall wage bill came mainly at the expense of the Ministries of Finance and Agriculture. The government of Zambia plans to reallocate resources—and the most recent MTEF (2006–2009) actually has fixed wage bill budget ceilings allocated to different sectors projected through three years, which was not the case in earlier years. In Zambia, the health and education sectors were allocated an increased share of the overall wage bill, and the Ministry of Finance, the Ministry of Constitutional and Statutory Expenditure, and the Electoral Commission of Zambia received considerable reductions.

Expanding the health wage bill is thought to lead to unsustainable growth in the overall wage bill. Analysis of aggregate civil service employment data as well as detailed simulations in Kenya and Zambia indicate that this outcome is not necessarily the case. The health sector on average accounts for about 10 percent of all public sector employees, according to the most recent aggregate data (figure 1.7). This finding suggests that expanding the health wage bill—through either increased hiring or increased salaries and allowances for health workers—in and of itself is likely to have only a small effect on the overall public sector wage bill. Moreover, if such changes apply only to doctors, the effect on the overall wage bill is likely to be very small, except in regions such as Eastern Europe and Central Asia and Latin America and the Caribbean, where doctors are more abundant. However, where the health sector is part of the civil service, wage increases or expanded hiring in the health sector could spill over into other sectors. This secondary spillover effect can be large.

Simulations illustrating the fiscal effect of increases in the health wage bill were carried out using information from two of the focus countries: Kenya and Zambia. For Kenya, only the direct effect was modeled, but for

Figure 1.7   Distribution of Civil Service Employees by Sector, 1996–2000

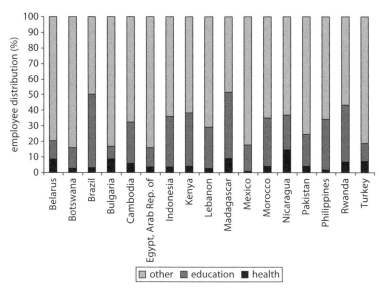

Source: World Bank Government Wages and Employment Dataset.

Zambia, the spillovers into the education sector were also modeled because data were available on the education wage bill and employment level.

These simulations show that the direct effect of increases in the health wage bill on the overall wage bill can be quite minimal. Suppose that in Zambia the wages of doctors or the number of doctors working in the public sector increased by 25 percent. This increase could be financed either through reallocating wage bill resources away from other sectors toward health or by expanding the overall public sector wage bill. If it were to be financed through reallocating wage bill resources, then the share of the overall wage bill going to the health sector would have to increase from 10.80 percent to 11.04 percent. If it were to be financed through additional overall wage bill resources, the overall wage bill would increase by 0.24 percent in real terms. Expanding the entire health work-force by 25 percent could be achieved by reallocating 2.70 percent of the overall public sector wage bill away from other sectors to health or by expanding the overall public sector wage bill by 2.70 percent in real terms. For Kenya, the direct effects are of similar magnitude.

In contrast, the indirect effect—when wage increases or expanded hiring spill over into other sectors—can be considerable. If the wage increase or expanded hiring in Zambia were to be financed through reallocation of wage bill resources to the education sector as well as to the health sector, this change would imply that 5.36 percent of wage bill resources would now need to be reallocated away from other sectors.[4] Similarly, if it were financed through additional overall wage bill resources, this change would imply an increase of 5.36 percent in the overall wage bill. Given that Zambia, compared with other countries, has a relatively small share of the wage bill devoted to the education sector (16.2 percent), this figure probably underestimates the average spillover effect across countries.

The simulations make clear that expanded hiring or increased wages in the health sector could easily be accommodated under certain conditions. GDP growth rates of 3 to 6 percent would be required to maintain a constant wage bill–to–GDP ratio in Kenya and Zambia if the health workforce were expanded by 25 percent (tables 1.3 and 1.4). If the spillover effects into other sectors—namely, education—could be avoided, only about 3 percent GDP growth would be required, well below the 6 to 9 percent that is projected through 2010 in Kenya (Kenya Ministry of Finance 2007) and the 6 to 7 percent projected in Zambia in the medium term (IMF 2007). Given that Kenya and Zambia are quite representative in terms of the size of the health sector relative to the public sector overall, the simulations are likely representative of other countries as well. Of course, as noted earlier, the governments of both Kenya and Zambia are trying to reduce the wage bill–to–GDP ratios quite substantially. But in countries with less contractionary overall wage bill policies, the increases in the overall wage bill that would result from expansion of the health workforce may be very fiscally tolerable.

Table 1.3   Impact on the Overall Public Sector Wage Bill of Staffing and Wages Changes in the Health Sector, Kenya

Scenario	Baseline: health wage bill/total wage bill (%)	New: health wage bill/total wage bill (%)	Increase (%)
Increase doctors' salaries by 25% (or increase number of doctors by 25%)	9.63	9.87	0.24
Increase nurses' salaries by 25% (or increase number of nurses by 25%)	9.63	10.82	1.19
Increase salaries for all health workers by 25% (or increase number of all health workers by 25%)	9.63	12.04	2.41

Source: World Bank staff calculations based on Kenya case study.

Table 1.4   Impact on the Overall Public Sector Wage Bill of Staffing and Wages Changes in the Health Sector, Zambia

Scenario	Baseline: health wage bill/total wage bill (%)	New: health wage bill/total wage bill (%)	Increase (%)
Increase doctors' salaries by 25% (or increase number of doctors by 25⁽	10.80	11.04	0.24
Increase nurses' salaries by 25% (or increase number of nurses by 25%	10.80	11.70	0.90
Increase salaries for all health workers by 25% (or increase number of all health workers by 25%)	10.80	13.50	2.70

Scenario	Baseline: education wage bill/total wage bill (%)	New: education wage bill/total wage bill (%)	Increase (%)
Increase teachers' salaries by 25 percent (or increase number of teachers by 25 percent)	12.38	15.04	2..66

Sources: World Bank staff calculations based on Zambia case study; World Bank 2006.

The Effect of the Wage Bill Budgeting Process on the Health Workforce

In the Dominican Republic, Kenya, and Zambia, the government reduced spending on the overall wage bill significantly, whereas in Rwanda spending remained fairly stable. In the Dominican Republic, Kenya, and Rwanda, the share of the overall wage bill going to the health sector increased steadily, indicating that the health sector was prioritized within the overall wage bill. In Zambia, this did not occur, but the delinking policy makes conclusions difficult to draw. What effect did these policies have on hiring in the health sector and on workforce levels?

In Kenya, the restrictive overall wage bill policy appears to have played a role in limiting the expansion of the health workforce. Despite the prioritization of the health sector within the overall wage bill, the number of staff members hired each year remained fairly constant. Evidence suggests significant unemployment exists among qualified health workers. About half of newly hired staff members in 2006 were unemployed before being hired. In 2006, there were about 10 applicants for every advertised job. The budget execution rate for the health wage bill is very high, with only a small number of funded vacancies that are not filled (table 1.5). This finding suggests that reductions in the overall wage bill

Table 1.5   Wage Bill Budget Execution Rates, 2004–07 (%)

Year	Dominican Republic	Kenya	Rwanda	Zambia
2004	95	101	99	—
2005	93	99	91	—
2006	107	—	91	50
2007	—	—	—	70

Source: Country case studies.

Note: Data included for available years; — = not available.

have created a fiscal constraint to scaling up the health workforce, at least in the short term. If more resources were available for the health wage bill, hiring could easily expand.

In Zambia, the impact on the health sector of the restrictive overall wage bill policy adopted in 2002 remains unclear. Currently, however, the main constraint to scaling up hiring in the short term is not fiscal. Clearly, the number of newly hired staff members within the Ministry of Health decreased significantly during the initial period of overall wage bill cuts beginning in 2002. However, this decrease was planned because staff was being delinked from the civil service during this period. In theory, no hiring at all was supposed to occur within the Ministry of Health, but in practice it did. No national data are available on the number of staff members hired by local boards of health (after delinking took place) beyond the staff members who were simply transferred from the central payroll. Information was collected for one board (in Lusaka), where 648 staff members (188 professional and 460 support staff members) were hired in addition to the more than 2,100 staff members absorbed from the Ministry of Health. This finding suggests that delinking the health sector from the civil service might have facilitated the expansion of the health workforce during the period of overall wage bill reductions, but the data needed to assess this hypothesis are simply not available. More recently, the boards of health were abolished, and staff members are now being relinked to the civil service.

According to the current MTEF, the number of health workers hired each year beyond those that are being reabsorbed—that is, new recruits— is projected to remain fairly stable. However, the government is having a hard time filling existing funded positions. Zambia has few unemployed health workers, and the budget execution rate for the health wage bill is only 70 percent in 2007. Those facts suggest that there is currently no fiscal constraint to scaling up the health workforce in Zambia. Additional wage bill resources are not needed to expand hiring in the health sector—additional candidates to hire are.

In Rwanda, the available evidence suggests that the overall wage bill policy did not create a fiscal constraint on scaling up the health workforce in the public sector. Data are not available on the number of newly hired staff members, but the stock of health workers in the public sector increased by more than 30 percent over a three-year period, suggesting that recruitment indeed took place. Budget execution rates for the health wage bill decreased since 2004, and few health workers are unemployed. Taken together, this information suggests that by prioritizing the health sector within a fairly flat overall wage bill, the government of Rwanda successfully scaled up the health workforce. The restrictive overall wage bill policy did not create a fiscal constraint for scaling up the health sector. The budget execution rate for the health wage bill was less than 100 percent, suggesting that lack of wage bill resources is not the main constraint to scaling up the health workforce.

In Rwanda, performance-based grants have relieved some of the upward pressure on the health wage bill resulting from health worker demands for increased salaries. Salaries of health workers employed in the public sector are counted as part of the overall wage bill. Performance-based grants are block grants and can be used to top up the salaries of health workers in the public sector. This portion is not counted as part of the wage bill. The grants were deliberately designed to give health facilities flexibility in appropriating the grant as deemed necessary, in return for meeting agreed-upon service delivery targets. Determining exactly what proportion of these grants is being used for salary top-ups is difficult. At the individual level, these top-ups sometimes increase a worker's salary by up to 86 percent. At the facility level, if only one-fourth of the grant was spent on salary top-ups (a conservative estimate, according to key informants), this amount would be sizable and would represent a considerable compensation increase for health workers.

In the Dominican Republic, the overall wage bill policy has not constrained hiring because expanding the health workforce in not a main priority for the government. Rather, growth in salary levels of health workers has been constrained, with important implications. In the Dominican Republic, hiring levels have decreased slightly, but staffing levels have remained fairly constant in recent years. As noted earlier, the Dominican Republic is different from the other three countries because the focus of its HRH strategy is not on scaling up. Workforce levels are quite high. Rather, increased resources for the health wage bill are used primarily to increase salaries and allowances of health workers in response to the demands of labor unions that are quite active in the country, as in the region generally. However, even with prioritizing health within the overall wage bill, the health wage bill has not been growing fast enough to meet the wage demands of labor unions. As a result, negotiations between the government and labor unions have shifted to include reductions in hours worked. The maximum hours worked stipulated in public sector contracts for health workers have decreased significantly; hours worked are now at 20 per week. This outcome is possible only because dual practice in the private sector is so prominent. With such a low level reached, future upward salary pressures are unlikely to be diffused through further decreases in hours worked. The Dominican Republic is a very interesting example of how overall wage bill policies have constrained growth in salary levels rather than in staffing. In turn, the fiscal constraint on increased salaries has led to reduced productivity of health workers in the public sector as they reduce hours worked.

In summary, the four country case studies clearly show that overall wage bill policies of the government have important implications for the health workforce when health workers are employed as part of the civil service. However, the consequences are by no means consistent across countries. In some settings, such as Rwanda and Zambia, existing wage bill resources are not fully spent, so the constraint on hiring more health workers—at least in the short term—is not primarily fiscal. Rather, the pool of health workers available to hire is insufficient, either because they simply are not there or because they are not willing to accept jobs in the public sector. In other settings, such as Kenya, existing wage bill resources are fully executed, health workers are available to hire, and an important fiscal constraint to scaling up the health workforce exists. In the Dominican Republic, fiscal constraints on the health wage bill led to reduced health worker productivity in public facilities. As shown in the next section, all of these countries have weaknesses in the administrative processes and public sector management functions. These, too, are important bottlenecks, hindering acceleration in hiring health workers in the public sector.

Managing Health Wage Bill Resources in the Public Sector

Although much attention is given at both the global and country levels to the need for increased spending on the health wage bill making sure that money is well spent is just as important for several reasons. First, the previous section makes clear that ministries of health could increase their influence on the wage bill allocation decision by demonstrating that additional wage bill resources would lead to better health service delivery outcomes for the population. Second, in situations where health wage bill resources are fixed and expansion of the health workforce will not occur, getting more for your money becomes a critical way to improve service delivery. Third, the inability of the ministry of health to fully execute the wage bill budget, despite critical shortages of health workers, implies that the health wage bill envelope is not the only constraint to scaling up the health workforce. Low budget execution rates suggest either a lack of available health workers to hire into funded positions or administrative bottlenecks in recruitment. The fact that the wage bill budget execution rate of the ministry of health in several of the focus countries is much lower than that of the ministry of education suggests capacity constraints that are particular to the ministry of health.

There is no standard measure of efficiency of the use of wage bill resources. Some key questions include the following: Are the available wage bill resources actually spent, and are health workers hired within a reasonable time frame? Are resources used to hire the right types of health workers (for example, skill mix),[5] and are they hired into the geographic areas where they are needed most? Is productivity high among health workers, and are they providing high-quality services? Do the incentives provided to health workers, including the method of remuneration, promote equitable geographic distribution, high productivity and quality of care, and low absenteeism?

This section draws primarily on the four country case studies. It focuses only on the following issues:

1. Policies and practices associated with some of the key human resource management functions in the public sector: recruiting health workers into funded positions, managing promotions, sanctioning, and executing transfers
2. Policies and practices related to the terms of work for health workers in the public sector, including remuneration
3. The role of these policies and practices in influencing selected health workforce outcomes: geographic distribution, absenteeism, and productivity.

The analysis of the basic human resource management functions provides a context for better understanding the efficiency issues associated with the use of the health wage bill. Through the examples provided in the four country case studies, the results of both good and bad management of these processes come to light. The discussion also establishes the foundation for the policy options discussed in this chapter's last section.

Recruitment of Health Workers in the Public Sector
All four country case studies demonstrate considerable delays in the recruitment process caused by the large number of actors involved. This process is one reason that the health wage bill budget is not fully executed. Considerable delays may occur in the hiring process because of the many steps involved, the large number of actors in different ministries, and insufficient capacity within each department (see, for example, Figure 2.8). Recruiting a health worker into the workforce in the public sector can take more than 13 months.

In all four country case studies, the recruitment process for health workers into the civil service usually involves other ministries and departments, which tend to play more central roles. Before someone can be recruited into a post, a funded vacancy needs to be created, which involves the creation or verification of the position within the ministry of health "establishment" and authorization for the funding of that position (see table 1.6). Both of these responsibilities often lie with agencies outside the health sector, although they are usually carried out in consultation with the ministry of health. In Kenya, the Public Service Commission is responsible for recruiting all civil servants, including health workers, after the positions have been funded. In Zambia, the Public Sector Management Division and the Management Development Division play this role, which allows the central authority to control the size of each line ministry's wage bill and, therefore, the overall public sector wage bill. The specific case studies in the subsequent chapters explain these processes in more detail.

In Kenya, Rwanda, and Zambia, the ministry of health *establishment* is the overall number of health workers that the government has determined is necessary to serve the country's population. It does not necessarily represent the number of health workers the government can employ. In many countries in Sub-Saharan Africa, particularly those that are modeled after the British civil service, the government will approve an establishment for each ministry. The establishment is based on both current staffing levels and long-term targets for scaling up in the future. The number of funded posts has to be within the limits of the approved establishment,

Table 1.6   Key Issues in Creation of Funded Posts

Country	Creation of funded posts
Dominican Republic	• No establishment (no strategic planning) exists. • The Office of Personnel Management is involved in approving all new positions.
Kenya	• The approved establishment is 42,154, of which 37,868 is funded. • Health workers are part of the overall civil service. • The Directorate of Personnel Management, in concert with the Treasury, approves all new positions.
Rwanda	• An establishment exists. • New positions are created during the MTEF process, providing greater flexibility in the creation of new posts.
Zambia	• The approved establishment is 51,040, of which 30,883 is funded. • Health workers are now part of the overall civil service. • The Public Sector Management Division, in concert with the Treasury, approves all new positions.

Source: Country case studies.

but not all the posts outlined in the establishment are necessarily funded. For example, in Kenya, 37,868 posts are funded out of a total establishment of 42,154. The establishment serves as a guideline and framework around which the ministry of health and civil service administration can negotiate the allocation of additional wage bill resources. The establishment is usually derived from health service delivery targets. For example, the establishment in Kenya was derived on the basis of a workload assessment for implementing the Kenya Essential Package of Health. In Zambia, the establishment was recently increased from 23,000 to 51,000 in accordance with normative staff-to-population ratios recommended by WHO.

The establishment provides a useful framework for wage bill budget negotiations in Kenya, Rwanda, and Zambia. Each year, through the wage bill budgeting process, the central authority approves funding for a certain number of additional posts within the establishment. The ministry of health does not have authority to change the establishment or to decide on how many additional posts within the establishment are filled. This power lies with the central authority. Nevertheless, the establishment is useful as a transparent tool and framework for human resource planning and for guiding negotiations between the ministry of health and the ministry of finance. Delays often occur, however, in the process of authorizing funding for posts within the establishment—again because of the many actors involved.

Posts in the establishment are usually specified by cadre, but they are not linked to any particular region. The establishment covers the ministry of health as a whole. The ministry of health, however, has full authority to link posts in the establishment to particular geographic locations and to link additional hiring to facilities with the highest needs. However, as will be discussed, this is usually not done.

The authority to recruit health workers into funded positions can rest either with the central ministry of health or with regional health authorities. In the case of the four countries examined in this report, recruitment is managed centrally for most types of workers. As the health wage bill budget is apportioned in the initial budgeting process, the central administration of recruitment ensures that new posts fall within the recognized allocations and overall establishment. However, this system can create large bottlenecks and bureaucratic delays in the ability of health facilities to fill vacancies in a timely manner (see table 1.7). It also makes strategic recruiting very difficult through the lack of flexibility in meeting the specific and varied needs of health facilities. Currently, no system is in place in several of the countries for allocating additional funded posts to the facilities where the staffing needs are greatest. The central authority is not positioned to be as responsive to local human resource issues. In some instances, once approval is received from the center, regional or district health officials are able to recruit from their own applicant pool. In other cases, they are not, and the central human resource authority for the health department assigns staff members. In certain decentralized settings, such as in Rwanda, local recruitment for certain cadres is permitted.

Table 1.7   Key Issues in Recruitment

Country	Recruitment
Dominican Republic	• Policy endorses regional management, but in practice most of the recruitment takes place at the central level. • Recruitment is not strategically planned.
Kenya	• Recruitment is centrally managed but not in a pooling mechanism. • Deployment is opaque. • Recruitment is characterized by long delays.
Rwanda	• Recruitment is both centrally and locally managed depending on the type of staff. • No pooling occurs.
Zambia	• Recruitment is centrally managed. • Recruitment is into a pool, and deployment to positions is not predetermined. • Recruitment is characterized by long delays.

Source: Country case studies.

The large number of steps required to fill a vacant post in the four country case studies leads to long delays. The specific recruiting process can vary somewhat from country to country; however, for the most part, the general process is similar. When a health facility or hospital sees the need to fill a post, whether the post is newly created or an existing vacancy, the facility makes a request to the district or regional health officials, who are then responsible for making a formal request to the ministry of health. If this request is approved, many times the ministry of health must then go to the civil service administration to match the post to an already established and funded position or to a newly funded position within the overall establishment. The official approval for recruitment to take place is then issued by the civil service administration. In many cases, the process is similar for filling newly funded positions as well as for recently vacated positions. For the latter, this process makes filling a gap and monitoring staffing levels accurately difficult, creating opportunities for ghost workers, as reported in several of the case studies. For instance, in Zambia, three officers are tasked with handling up to 900 requests for filling recently vacated positions. In Kenya, the agency responsible for recruitment for the entire civil service—about 190,000 employees—consists of only 38 employees: 20 secretaries, 10 clerical officers, and 8 officers. In many instances, skilled health workers are a scarce commodity, and these delays add to the problems of hiring, training, and retaining health workers in the public sector.

In some cases, the method of matching staff members to vacant positions does not promote retention of health workers in remote areas. Candidates can be selected either through a central pooling process or by recruitment for specific, predefined positions. In cases where the ministry of health recruits a pool of candidates and then assigns individuals to various vacant positions, the location where a health worker is posted is not necessarily strategic. Evidence shows that by matching an advertised position to specific posts, applicants are more likely to self-select and therefore are less likely to abscond (Dussault and Franceschini 2006; Serneels and others 2006). Additionally, a health worker applies to a general pool without any prior knowledge of where he or she may be posted. For example, in Zambia, the Ministry of Health places one advertisement at the start of the fiscal year that lists only the types of positions for which it is recruiting, without any detail on numbers or locations. This procedure often leads to rejection of the assignment if the health worker is posted to an unfavorable location or to absenteeism. This outcome might have contributed to the situation in Zambia where the government was unable to fill all funded positions. In 2007, the Ministry of Health in Zambia received Treasury authority to recruit 1,700 health workers, but it was able to effectively fill only 1,300 of those positions. In addition, the central pooling and deployment of health workers can be perceived as being opaque and prone to corruption and may contribute to regional inequities in health worker staffing levels. In Rwanda, facilities have the authority to hire certain cadres of staff locally, making posts easier to fill and staff members easier to retain.

Overall, the recruitment process in the four countries is not timely and is not targeted to areas with the highest need for staff. First is the fact that the process usually involves several steps across various levels of government, thus leading to delays in filling positions. The situation is worse when a preexisting position needs to be filled because of the transfer or retirement of a worker. In several countries, the same process applies, resulting in gaps, interruptions in service provision, or—worse still—continuous payments by the central government against a vacant position (payments for a ghost worker). Second, often the central government manages recruitment and may not be familiar with the particular needs of the local facilities. If not strategically implemented, this distancing of the recruitment process from the point of service may lead to inequitable and inefficient distribution of health workers. Third, by recruiting into a central pool rather than into predefined positions, the process of deploying the workers to various locations—some considered more favorable than others—risks being perceived as opaque. This method also does not take advantage of different preferences among health workers for different positions that can be harnessed to improve retention. For example, in Kenya, the Ministry of Health moved from recruiting into an overall pool and then deploying workers as needed to using a system where recruitment was tied to specific posts that applicants were made aware of before applying through the Emergency Hiring Program. The result of this policy change was improved allocation, and when surveyed three months later, workers expressed intent to remain in their assigned posts.

Managing Promotions, Sanctioning, and Transfers

More strategic management of promotions and transfers in the four country case studies can affect the geographic distribution of workers. Promotions and transfers depend in large part on a vacant position becoming available, although sometimes they could be automatic and linked to tenure. The processes of transfer and promotion are prone to bureaucratic delays similar to those associated with filling a new post (table 1.8).

As with recruitment, promotion authority can rest at the center and therefore depend on effective communication and responsiveness from various levels of government and, in some cases, other line ministries, such as the public service commission or the civil service administration. This process leads to the same delays experienced in the recruitment process. In several cases, where flexibility in the ability to provide promotions was limited, delays were experienced, and promotion was often based on seniority rather than performance. This factor is often at odds with stated human resource policies, which tout performance as their major criterion for promotion.

In Zambia, salaries follow people. When a position is funded, the payments are made against the person in question, and this funding continues to accrue to the person regardless of where he or she moves within the country. Thus, if the person is transferred to a different district, a vacant post is not necessarily created by that departure. In Rwanda, salaries follow the post and not the person; therefore, if a person leaves a post, the funding for a replacement is assured because the vacated

Table 1.8   Key Issues in Promotions and Transfers

Countries	Promotions and transfers
Dominican Republic	• Promotions are supposed to be based on a performance evaluation system, but it has never been fully implemented. • Promotions are based primarily on seniority and political favoritism. • Transfers into the capital are prohibited.
Kenya	• Promotion policy follows the overall civil service system. • Promotion process is often delayed, resulting in low morale among health workers. Attempts at reform are in the process but have yet to be implemented.
Rwanda	• Promotions are supposed to be based on a performance evaluation system; however, evidence shows that this system is not always followed. • Allowances do not promote effective distribution of health workers. • A funded and vacant position has to be available in another facility for a transfer to occur.
Zambia	• Promotions and transfers are based on a vacant position becoming available. • The process is plagued by bureaucratic delays.

Source: Country case studies.

position is funded. This system also ensures that movements occur only when a funded post elsewhere is available and reduces the inequitable distribution of health workers that could arise if several people moved away from remote locations to more favorable places.

The Dominican Republic strictly manages transfers to maintain geographic balance in staffing levels. For example, transfers to the capital, Santo Domingo, are prohibited, whereas transfers out of the capital city to other provinces are strongly encouraged.

All four countries have formal legislation governing the termination and sanctioning of civil service employees, but the formal policy can be very different from the actual practice (see table 1.9). Given the persistence of absenteeism in many countries, the policies for termination and sanctioning are not adequately enforced. Limited data are available on absenteeism, however, because of the difficulty in distinguishing between legitimate reasons for absenteeism, such as training and visiting other facilities to provide care, and other causes, such as moonlighting during working hours, absconding, or taking unauthorized leave.

Sanctions are rarely enforced, often because of the scarcity of workers and the resulting difficulty in replacing them. Moreover, disciplinary action for technical issues often rests with the professional councils, which tend to be lenient with their own cadres. However, in a 2006 survey of health facilities in Zambia, of a total of 300 staff members that left their jobs, 8 percent were either dismissed or suspended.

Weak sanctioning and termination mechanisms tend to disproportionately affect those who need services the most because replacing workers in the areas with most need is more difficult. Hence, the already weak health service delivery system is perpetuated.

Table 1.9   Key Issues in Termination and Sanctioning

Countries	Termination and sanctioning
Dominican Republic	• Policy is in place but not followed. • No evidence exists of termination or severe sanctioning occurring.
Rwanda	• There are two levels of sanctioning. One can be done at the facility level, and the second is conducted through the Civil Service Commission.
Zambia	• Terminations follow civil service statutes. • Terminations do occur, but not necessarily strategically, because absenteeism still persists.

Source: Country case studies.

Terms of Employment for Health Workers in the Public Sector

In the four focus countries, health workers in the public sector are primarily employed as civil servants (see table 1.10). Thus, they are subject to the general statutes, regulations, and laws governing the rest of the civil service.

Health workers in the public sector in the country case studies are employed mainly on permanent contracts. More than 90 percent of health workers in Kenya and more than three-fourths of health workers in the Dominican Republic are employed on permanent contracts. Permanent contracts are the primary mode of employment in the public sector in general.

Use of permanent contracts has important implications. First, such contracts are intended to enhance professionalism and integrity of civil servants by protecting them from arbitrary and nontransparent personnel actions (for example, firing without just cause and corruption in hiring). But the trade-off is that permanent contracts also reduce the ability of managers to ensure that staff members focus their efforts on performance because tenure protections make disciplinary actions (particularly, dismissals) more difficult. This situation poses an unavoidable trade-off between depoliticized management of civil servants and staff performance (facilitated by giving managers greater discretion over how they motivate their staff) (Klingner and Nalbandian 2002; Reid 2005). Second, hiring staff on permanent contracts creates long-term contingent liabilities for the government in the form of salary and pension payments.

Table 1.10   Key Issues in Tenure Policies

Countries	Tenure policies
Dominican Republic	• Most workers are part of overall civil service. • Short-term contracts are used more than government regulations and policies allow.
Kenya	• Most workers are part of the overall civil service. • Short-term contractual employment is limited. • The Emergency Hiring Program is used to circumvent restrictive contracting processes and inefficiencies still in the system.
Rwanda	• Most workers are part of the overall civil service. • Current reforms aimed at delinking health workers from civil service and having them employed by facilities.
Zambia	• Most workers are part of the overall civil service. • The government unsuccessfully attempted to delink health workers from the overall civil service. • Use of short-term or contractual employment is minimal.

Source: Country case studies.

The use of temporary contracts can help overcome delays in the hiring process and match the length of service to available funding, but their use remains fairly limited in the four country studies. Various approaches can be used to circumvent the difficulties and lack of flexibility of hiring health workers in the overall civil service. In many countries, short-term contracts are used to expedite hiring, to increase flexibility for the government to adjust to fiscal conditions, and to hire health workers using operational budgets to avoid wage bill restrictions. The use of short-term contracts is often limited to strategic purposes such as effectively and rapidly scaling up the workforce in certain instances where recruitment and contracting inefficiencies would have caused significant delays. For example, the Kenya Emergency Hiring Program used short-term contracts to hire staff members outside the normal recruitment process. Health workers' expectations need to be managed, however, because contractual workers often expect to be integrated into the regular and pensionable civil service. Implicit agreements to do so often exist. A second approach is removing the health sector from the civil service and hiring health workers on contracts, as in Zambia. The health boards, which were to have taken up service delivery responsibilities, had separate conditions of service (often better), which would not have been possible if the workers were part of the civil service.

The fact that health workers are employed primarily as civil servants in the four country studies has important implications for salary levels. In the Dominican Republic, Kenya, and Rwanda, health worker salaries are based on a uniform civil service pay scale; thus, adjusting health worker salary levels without affecting salaries of all civil servants is difficult. For a doctor or nurse to receive a pay increase, the rest of the government workers who are at the same level would have to receive the same increase. Such increases can become both politically and fiscally impossible, especially if the wage bill ceiling and other fiscal constraints are significant. In Zambia, a separate civil service pay scale has been created just for the health sector. It allows remuneration to be increased only for health workers, which can be pivotal in both recruiting and retaining health workers. This system also avoids problems of comparison across sectors and the need to negotiate with other civil service employees. In those cases where health workers have been delinked entirely (for example, the experience in Zambia with the boards of health), health workers are not civil servants, and remuneration is based on the budget envelope and salary scales determined by the autonomous health management units.

Allowances are an important part of remuneration for individual health workers and account for a significant part of the health wage bill in the four countries. Nevertheless, allowances are often not used strategically. The total wage bill is usually a combination of the base salary, the allowances, and other incentives paid to the health worker. In many countries, allowances constitute a large part of the total wages. For instance, allowances account for 45 percent of the overall health wage bill in Kenya and 14 percent of the overall wage bill in the Dominican Republic. Some of the more common allowances include housing, rural, risk, on-call, uniform, overtime, and retention payments. Not only are allowances important financially because of their size, but also they can be used strategically to alleviate labor market inequities and to provide strong incentives for increasing performance. For example, if used strategically, allowances can adjust for hardship experienced by doctors practicing in rural or conflict areas. However, in most cases they are effective salary top-ups that are not always used in a transparent or effective manner.[6] In Kenya, for instance, the more lucrative housing allowance that accrues to residents in the Nairobi area has created a disincentive for workers to locate in remote areas. In the Dominican Republic, after a worker leaves a location, the geographic allowance turns into a permanent component of the worker's wage, contrary to the stated policy. This situation generates distortions in the objectives of the allowance and generates significant upward pressure on the budget because people keep claiming these allowances even after leaving the relevant position.

An interesting example of strategic use of allowances occurs in Rwanda. Allowances are partially tied to performance. Performance-based grants are provided to facilities according to an agreed set of performance benchmarks. These grants (at least 40 percent of total wages) are used to pay salary top-ups. Because this policy has only recently been implemented, the effect on service delivery and staff performance is not yet known.

Remuneration in general can affect productivity, geographic distribution, and efficiency of the health workforce (see table 1.11). The effect of remuneration on staffing outcomes was not assessed in great detail in the four country case studies. However, the evidence from the literature shows that alternative remuneration methods—especially when performance based—can increase productivity and quality of care and improve retention (see appendix D). In addition, strategic use of allowances can help address geographic imbalances by increasing the amount paid to those who work in areas with the most need, but such allowances often must be accompanied by nonfinancial incentives (Dussault and Franceschini 2006).

Table 1.11   Key Issues in Remuneration

Country	Remuneration
Dominican Republic	• Large regional variation exists in salaries. • Allowances differ from those set out in policy. A lot of discretion exists in how allowances are paid, even among health workers in the same cadre. • Allowances are not used strategically. • Unions play a large role in salary negotiations.
Kenya	• Health workers are part of civil service pay scale. • Casual employees are paid through local revenues, from user fees, or from operational budgets. • Allowances are widely used, accounting for 45% of total health wage bill. • Allowances are not used strategically. • Allowance leakage problems exist.
Rwanda	• Salaries are tied to posts and not to employees. • Salaries are based on an index system. • Allowances have been used to circumvent the civil service pay scale. • The share of allowances relative to total remuneration has been decreasing over time. • Performance-based bonuses are used to provide top-ups for good performance.
Zambia	• Doctors and other health workers have distinct salary scales, separate from the overall civil service pay scale. • Administrative workers in the health sector are paid on the overall civil service pay scale. • Allowances are not captured in the overall wage bill. • Allowances are not strategic.

Source: Country case studies.

In summary, the analysis has shown that there are large inefficiencies in how governments allocate and manage their health wage bill resources. Evidence shows that many of the focus countries are not able to fully use their current health wage bill resources. For example, in 2007, Zambia's health wage bill execution rate was only 70 percent. The inability to fully execute the wage bill can be attributed in large part to capacity constraints within the government as well as to processes that are complicated, involve several governmental departments and levels of administration, and are plagued by delays. Recruitment is often centrally managed and not strategic. People are not always posted to the places of greatest need, in part because of the way recruitment is done. Candidates often apply to a central pool rather than for specific positions and are then deployed, which contributes to higher attrition rates.

The country case studies also show that the lack of autonomy over key functions is one of the factors limiting the strategic use of health wage bill resources. For functions over which the ministry of health has a high degree of autonomy, limited capacity and the fact that policies are simply not followed are the main factors limiting strategic use of wage bill resources.

Policy Options to Address Fiscal Constraints on the Health Wage Bill and to Improve Management of the Health Workforce in the Public Sector

Governments might consider several policy options to address the fiscal constraints to expanding the health wage bill (where they arise) and to improve key human resource management policies and practices that affect how health wage bill resources are used. The remainder of this chapter discusses these policy options. They are not intended as prescriptive recommendations, nor is the evidence supporting each policy option fully summarized. Rather, the challenges and the enabling and inhibiting factors for success associated with each policy option are discussed at some length to identify where each policy option may be most appropriate. Some of these policy options require significant public sector reform, with considerable risk. Others are more conservative and can be implemented rapidly within the existing administrative environment. The following policy options are discussed in this section:

- Strengthening accountability and improving human resource management capacity within the ministry of health
- Using allowances more strategically and using payment mechanisms other than salary
- Improving the predictability of health wage bill budgets
- Enhancing the position of the ministry of health in the wage bill budget negotiation process
- Easing the fiscal constraints on the overall wage bill
- Making better use of donor assistance for health
- Transferring control of certain human resource management functions to the ministry of health while keeping the health workforce within the civil service
- Decentralizing certain human resource management functions to the local level
- Removing the health workforce from the civil service and the overall wage bill

Strengthening Accountability

Lines of accountability could be strengthened, the information base could be improved, and capacity within the ministry of health could be strengthened to bring current human resource management practices more in line with stated policies. A remarkable finding across all the country studies is that many human resource management policies are not followed. The country studies did not examine the reasons for this finding in any great detail, but some emerging issues point to potential policy responses. First, the incentives to adhere to policies could be strengthened. They are currently weak partly because the existing budgeting process for the health wage is not based on service delivery or health workforce performance and partly because promotion and sanctioning policies for managers are often not fully implemented.

Second, processes related to many human resource management functions could be made more transparent. Some indications from the country case studies are that the processes related to many human resource management functions are opaque and vulnerable to corruption. Strong evidence from the literature indicates that transparent, meritocratic recruitment and selection procedures within the public sector contribute significantly to worker productivity (Anderson, Reid, and Ryterman 2003; Rauch and Evans 2000; Recanatini, Prati, and Tabellini 2005).

Third, capacity to carry out basic functions could be strengthened. Greater automation of data and record keeping would greatly reduce processing times for many human resource management functions. In many countries, data entry and record keeping are still done manually. Accurate data how many workers are employed in the public sector and where they are working are not available in a timely manner. A review of civil service reform experiences has shown that strengthening human resource information systems is relatively easy to implement compared with other reforms (box 1.1). One of the key success factors of the Kenya Emergency Hiring Program is that recruitment was managed through a computerized, just-in-time system with regular monitoring of staff. The time to fill a post was half that required for routine civil service recruitment.

Using Allowances More Strategically

Where the ministry of health has autonomy, allowances could be used much more strategically, and alternatives to salary payment could be considered to strengthen the incentives for good performance. The

Box 1.1

Challenges of Civil Service and Administrative Reform

The World Bank recently released a report examining its support to countries in the field of public sector reform in four areas: public financial management, tax administration, transparency, and civil service reform (World Bank 2008). The analysis shows that lending usually improved performance for the first three themes but failed to do so in the case of civil service reform. These findings highlight the extreme difficulty in implementing civil service reform, because of the large fiscal impact, its highly politicized nature, and opposition from heavily vested interests.

Civil service and administrative (CSA) reform involves all aspects of the management and organization of personnel. World Bank programs in this area included reforms to the personnel information system (including civil service censuses); to the overall size of the civil service; to career paths, pay grades (decompression), and other aspects of the incentive system; and to the organization of ministries. The reforms are evaluated against outcomes that include a civil service that attracts, retains, and motivates competent staff; a transparent, nondiscretionary pay regime appropriate to local labor market conditions; a wage bill within overall budgetary constraints; reduced salary compression and turnover; and interministerial coordination.

The report found that World Bank–supported CSA reforms were unsatisfactory in most cases. Many times, the general motivation of World Bank involvement evolved from a need to address the issue of an affordable wage bill as a significant component of public sector expenditures. As a result, CSA reforms often emphasized retrenchment and salary decompression, overlooking the politically unrealistic nature of these actions and assuming without evidence that these changes would bring about improved public administration. Given the recognition of relative failure in focusing on wage bill containment issues alone, the World Bank has shifted its focus to human resource management reform. These reforms include merit-based recruitment and promotion to increase efficiency of current wage bill resources and to improve overall civil service functions. Successful reforms were attributed to the following factors: analytical diagnosis and advice, pragmatic opportunism in selecting reforms to support, realistic expectations from the donor community, appropriate packages of lending instruments, tangible indicators of success, and effective donor coordination. Although the success factors are meant to pertain to overall civil service reform, they can easily be related to reform efforts within the health sector workforce.

(continued)

Box 1.1 *(Continued)*

The accompanying table summarizes the areas of CSA reform that are more or less feasible, depending on fiscal, political, or capacity constraints. Training is the most feasible option and thus shows the most success. Downsizing, compensation reforms, human resource management reforms, organizational reforms, and demand-side reforms each are more difficult.

Areas of Civil Service and Administrative Reform

Component	Political risk	Financial cost	Demanding of capacity?	Countries that successfully implemented reforms	Countries showing little or no progress
Pay and employment data	Minimal	Modest	Yes—but capacity building is part of project	Guyana, Rep. of Yemen	Honduras, Uganda
Downsizing	High	Significant one-time costs for retrenchment	Yes, to do it right (targeted)	India, Russian Fed., Tanzania	Bulgaria, Cambodia, Ethiopia, Guyana, Sri Lanka, Uganda, Rep. of Yemen
Compensation reforms	High	Yes	Yes	Albania, Bulgaria	Guyana, Indonesia, Rep. of Yemen
Human resource management reforms	High	Moderate	Yes	Albania, Bolivia (pilots), Bulgaria	Ghana

Source: World Bank 2008.

remuneration methods in the four country case studies are very similar and focus on salary and nonperformance-based allowances. In Rwanda, a performance-based allowance has recently been introduced, but it is too early to measure the effect on health workforce performance.

The available evidence from the literature suggests that allowances could be used more strategically. For the allowances that apply to all civil servants and that are not within the ministry of health's control, reforms might not be possible. But allowances within the control of the health sector should be used to provide stronger incentives for performance.

Appendix D summarizes some of the key findings related to performance-based allowances—at both the individual and facility levels—and other alternative payment mechanisms for health workers.

International experience shows that alternatives to salary payment can be a very effective way of improving health workforce performance in the public sector (see appendix D for a review of the evidence). Nevertheless, reforms such as performance-based pay require careful selection of the indicators on which performance will be measured and careful design of incentives so that they align health worker behavior with the goals of the health system. Many countries, such as Rwanda, have experimented with performance-based pay, and their experiences make clear that monitoring capacity, management capacity, and a flexible institutional and legal framework are important factors for success.

Improving the Predictability of the Health Wage Bill

Within the current budgeting process, the predictability of the health wage bill could be improved by budgeting for a longer period. If the previous reforms are not suitable, then at minimum the wage bill budget for the health sector could be determined for a longer period. In all the country case studies, recruitment planning suffered significant constraints because of the uncertainty of the health wage bill budget. In most of the countries, the wage bill budget is given for a one- to three-year period, yet staff members are hired on permanent contracts. Moreover, in some of the country case studies, the health wage bill budget was not set until well into the fiscal year, leaving little time to recruit staff members, partly explaining low budget execution rates. These significant planning challenges could be partially addressed if wage bill budgets covered longer periods. Of course, the obvious challenge with this policy option is that government revenues and expenses are difficult to predict (for example, economic shocks, natural disasters, and elections may intervene).

Enhancing the Negotiation Position of the Ministry of Health

The position of the ministry of health in wage bill budget negotiations could be strengthened so that an increasing share of the overall wage bill is devoted to the health sector. If the overall wage bill is fixed and the health workforce remains part of the civil service, then the only way to increase the health wage bill is to allocate existing or additional wage bill resources away from other sectors toward health. To receive such resources, the ministry of health needs to improve its negotiation strategy. The health sector competes with other sectors for additional wage bill resources. The country analysis makes clear that although countries often have a policy that prioritizes the health sector within the overall wage bill, in practice this priority is not always given.

The ministry of health could play a more active role in the budget negotiation process in two ways. First, it could ensure that stated national development policies are adhered to and are reflected in wage bill budget allocations. Second, it could create HRH strategies that clearly make the case for why additional wage bill resources ought to be devoted to the health sector. This activity involves moving beyond the traditional focus in national HRH strategies of estimating long-term staffing needs to a much more incremental, short-term, results-based approach. It is important for the ministry of health to identify priority short-term actions for incremental resources and to try to demonstrate the likely effect on health service delivery of these actions. Such HRH strategies are rare, but a good example of such a practice occurs in Zambia, where three fully costed incremental scenarios were put forth with the effect on service delivery outlined.

Several factors inhibit creating results-based HRH strategies. The first factor is the current wage bill budgeting process. In many countries, it does not provide the incentives for developing such HRH strategies. The health wage bill is not within the control of the ministry of health and is unpredictable. Thus, the ministry has no incentive to plan something it cannot control. This situation leads to weak plans, weak negotiating positions, and fewer wage bill resources, thereby reducing further the incentive to be strategic—resulting in a state of low-level equilibrium.

The second inhibiting factor is the very weak evidence base on different health workforce policies available and their effect on outcomes. Agencies such as WHO, the World Bank, the Capacity Project, and the Global Health Workforce Alliance need to support the creation of a global evidence base for health workforce policies that countries can access.

The third inhibiting factor is weak monitoring and evaluation systems. At a minimum, the ministry of health should collect accurate information on how many health workers are employed in the public sector, where they are working, and where the areas of highest staffing need are located. Constantly monitoring the effect of policy reforms is also important so that the results produced by additional wage bill resources (for example, from last year's budget negotiation cycle) can be demonstrated.

Developing HRH strategies with the budget negotiation cycle in mind would go a long way in improving position of the position of the ministry of health. It could help change the perception that is often held by the ministry of finance and cabinet that devoting more resources to the health wage bill is not the best use of scarce budgetary resources.

Easing the Fiscal Constraints

The fiscal constraint on the overall wage bill could be relaxed to accommodate expansion of the health wage bill. This option entails a shift in fiscal policy of the government, either to relax overall wage bill ceilings or to relax limits on the fiscal deficit. This shift may require minimal reforms in some countries, but in others it may require changes to budget laws. Under this policy option, the ministry of health would take a more active role in trying to influence the overall wage bill policy of the government, arguing that the fiscal impact on the overall wage bill resulting from expanding the health workforce is outweighed by the benefits it brings to the population. One important enabling factor is that the overall wage bill may not need to increase much to finance an expanded health wage bill, as shown in the earlier simulations.

This policy option should be considered only in certain settings. As noted earlier, a strong economic rationale exists for controlling the size of the overall wage bill. In the absence of strong evidence on what level would be "too high" and would bring about negative macroeconomic consequences, governments are likely to rely on regional or global comparisons. Thus, in countries with above average wage bill spending levels (relative to both government spending and GDP), this policy option may not be suitable. But even in countries with low levels of spending on the overall wage bill, this policy option is fraught with several challenges. First, the ministry of health may have difficulty influencing the overall wage bill policy because the ministry is usually not even part of the decision-making body that sets the policy. Second, a very strong case would need to be made for how additional wage bill resources would improve service delivery and health outcomes of the population. To achieve such outcomes, ministries of health need health workforce strategies that have very clear short-term and medium-term priorities, are based on sound evidence, are costed, and clearly show what the effect would be of increasing the overall wage bill to finance incremental hiring or wage increases in the health sector. As the analysis has shown, examples of good practices exist (such as the HRH strategy in Zambia), but not in most developing countries.

Making Better Use of Donor Assistance

By working with international agencies, governments could reduce the volatility and unpredictability of donor assistance for health, thus allowing governments to devote more donor assistance for health to remuneration of health workers. Two recent developments have triggered increased interest in this policy option. First, donor assistance for health has increased substantially in developing countries in recent years (Gottret and Schieber 2006). Second, health workforce capacity has been increasingly identified as one of the main constraints to scaling up health service delivery in developing countries, and several donor agencies have stated their commitment to addressing this challenge. The obvious advantage of using donor assistance for health is that it is a significant source of health financing in developing countries (Gottret and Schieber 2006). But several significant challenges are associated with this policy option.

First, a mismatch exists between the length of time for which donors commit funding and the current terms of work in the public sector. As the country studies show, health workers in the public sector are currently hired primarily on permanent contracts. Yet donor assistance for health is short term, unpredictable, and volatile (Gottret and Schieber 2006). On the donor side, this situation might be resolved by making longer-term commitments. For example, recently in Malawi, the U.K. Department for International Development provided resources to increase health workers' salaries significantly over a six-year period. From the government's side, alternative contracting arrangements should be explored to make financing salaries with donor aid easier. The Emergency Hiring Program in Kenya (box 1.2) is a good example where health workers paid through donor resources were hired on three-year contracts to match donor commitments.

Second, the current modality of donor aid is not conducive to using resources to hire health workers. When donor aid for health is provided as general budget support and flows directly to the ministry of finance, resources can be channeled by the government to the health wage bill and can be used to expand hiring or increase salaries of health workers in the public sector. But experience has shown that aid fungibility is an important risk through this modality. A large portion of aid is provided off budget and cannot be used to hire health workers in the public sector (Gottret and Schieber 2006).

Third, donor aid is often earmarked for specific purposes—often disease related—restricting what types of health workers can be hired through

Box 1.2

The Kenya Emergency Hiring Program: A Promising Practice in Using Donor Assistance to Scale Up the Health Workforce

Donor resources have been used successfully to scale up recruitment, and many of the negative consequences associated with using external resources to pay salaries have been avoided. Beginning in 2006, donors worked with the Ministry of Health to develop an Emergency Hiring Program (EHP) to address staffing shortages in underserved areas. Under this program, the U.S. President's Emergency Plan for AIDS Relief; the Global Fund to Fight AIDS, Tuberculosis, and Malaria; and the Clinton Foundation provided resources to support hiring of health workers on three-year contracts tied to specific geographic areas. The EHP substantially affected the fiscal space for hiring health workers in the public sector. In 2006, recruitment of health workers in the public sector increased dramatically—triple the number in previous years—with the majority of hiring (83 percent) funded by donors through the EHP. Under the EHP, funds are provided to the government, and the staff is employed by the Ministry of Health. Salaries and allowances are set at the same levels as those of health workers in the Ministry of Health. Because staff members are hired on short-term contracts, no contingent wage bill liability is created for the government. The government has indicated that it intends to have the necessary wage bill resources after three years to absorb the additional staff, but it has made no formal agreement of commitment. Essentially, the donors have bought time for the government to raise the necessary wage bill resources.

In addition, the recruitment process under the EHP was computerized, and recruitment authority was delegated from the Public Service Commission to the Ministry of Health. Short-listing 2,600 health staff from a total 7,000 applicants took only 10 days. The first successful recruits were in their posts fewer than five months after the jobs were advertised, considerably faster than the 13 months the traditional recruitment process sometimes takes.

Source: Kenya case study (chapter 2).

those funds. This condition sometimes prevents the use of donor aid for hiring health workers who deliver a broad range of services.

Fourth, if donor assistance for health is not well coordinated, it has the potential to generate wage differentials across different employers, resulting in unintended movements of health workers across employers or service delivery units. In Ethiopia, for example, a review of the Global

Fund to Fight AIDS, Tuberculosis, and Malaria (GFATM) experience suggested that jobs in HIV-related services became more attractive after GFATM resources became available (Banteyerga, Kidanu, and Stillman 2006). A recent analysis of wages in several countries found that government salaries did not match those in the donor and nongovernmental sector (McCoy and others 2008).

The country case studies did not analyze the use of donor funding to support the expansion of the health workforce in great depth. However, the Emergency Hiring Program in Kenya exemplifies good practices in addressing many of the challenges in using donor assistance for health to scale up the health workforce in the public sector (box 1.2). In addition, an analysis of the policies and practices of funding health worker remuneration using grants from two major donor agencies—GFATM and the Global Alliance for Vaccines and Immunization (GAVI)—are summarized in appendix E, with the main points described in box 1.3.

Transferring Authority over Human Resource Functions

Subject to certain conditions, authority over selected HRH functions could be transferred to the ministry of health, while the health wage bill was retained within the overall wage bill. If some of the enabling conditions are not present or autonomy over all functions is not necessary, then an alternative is to grant the ministry of health autonomy over only certain functions. Depending on the extent of autonomy, this policy

---

Box 1.3

Summary of Policies and Practices in GFATM and GAVI HSS for Remuneration of Health Workers

GFATM and GAVI—two agencies examined for this report—have quite flexible policies toward funding health worker remuneration; however, a key condition is sustainability. The GFATM guidelines for Round 7 proposals say that human resources for health activities will be funded if a strong link between the proposed activities and health systems strengthening (HSS) as well as the three target diseases can be demonstrated. The GAVI HSS guidelines highlight health workforce mobilization, distribution, and motivation related to immunization and other health services as one of three major priority areas for funding. The guidelines state that sustainability of these expenditures when GAVI HSS funds are no longer available must be demonstrated.

Box 1.3 *(Continued)*

Remuneration methods for frontline health workers are different under the GAVI and GFATM grants and suggest differences in the effect on the health workforce. Within GAVI, the remuneration payments to frontline health workers are mostly in the form of allowances. Within GFATM, however, most of the remuneration to frontline health workers is in the form of salaries. This difference suggests that GAVI HSS grants focus more on supplementing the income and improving the performance of the current health workforce, whereas GFATM grants focus more on creating newly funded positions, thereby expanding the health workforce.

Some emerging evidence indicates wage distortions in some countries; however, further work is needed in this area. In Ethiopia, for example, a review of the GFATM experience suggested that jobs in HIV-related services became more attractive after GFATM resources became available. In Benin, evidence indicates that facilities supported through GFATM grants followed the government pay scale and had just as much trouble attracting staff members as government facilities. Very little labor movement out of government facilities occurred. A recent analysis of wages in several countries found that government salaries did not match those in the donor and nongovernmental sector.

Within GFATM and GAVI HSS, sustainability issues surrounding payment of salaries and allowances to frontline health workers are not adequately addressed. Sustainability issues can be dealt with in several ways. Health workers who are paid salaries can be hired on short-term contracts. Allowances can be paid during the time of the grants only. The government can also commit to take over payment of salaries of newly hired staff members or to pay allowances when grant funding runs out. More than half of GFATM Round 6 grants assume that the government will absorb the salary and allowance payments at the end of the grant period, but there is no explicit agreement from the government to do so. Within GAVI as well, the issue of sustainability is not dealt with adequately.

Source: Appendix E.

option may or may not entail removing health workers from the civil service. For example, if the main issue is that the ministry of health salary scale is too compressed or salaries are too low, then the health sector can be granted its own salary scale within the civil service, as is the case currently in Zambia. In Kenya, the increased autonomy given to the ministry of health over the recruitment process significantly reduced the time required to fill a vacancy and improved retention significantly, but only because significant capacity building took place within the ministry before the policy reform. In Rwanda, the ministry of health designed and implemented a performance-based allowance scheme that is being used to supplement health workers' salaries. This change was possible partly because of strong monitoring and evaluation capacity within the ministry of health.

Decentralizing

Subject to certain conditions—including adequate human resource management capacity—key human resource management functions could be transferred from the central level to the local level. Given that in all four country case studies, health workers were employed by the central government, the case studies do not provide rich evidence on the effect of decentralization. However, appendix C summarizes the evidence from the literature on how decentralizing functions within the health sector affects selected outcomes of human resources for health.

The main rationale for transferring certain functions to local units is to improve administrative and allocative efficiency. In terms of administrative efficiency, allowing local recruitment could shorten the time to fill a position, eliminating the many steps involved in obtaining central-level approval. It could also lead to a better match of candidates with the appropriate position, because the final selection of candidates would be done locally. This outcome was clearly demonstrated by the Emergency Hiring Program in Kenya. Similarly, letting local units set salaries and allowances allows them to take into account local labor market conditions. For example, salaries for certain areas may need to be much higher to attract staff members, but common national pay scales may prevent such local discretion.

Potential challenges also exist. Without adequate oversight and monitoring, allowing local hiring and firing may increase the likelihood of corruption and nepotism. Decentralizing wage setting could exacerbate geographic inequities if wealthier provinces are able to pay higher wages. It might also lead to wage inflation, as districts and provinces compete for scarce staff. Moreover, sufficient capacity is needed at the local level to carry out key functions. Interestingly, in Rwanda, the central government had lower execution rates (80 percent) than the local government (101 percent) before decentralization, but after decentralization this trend was reversed, with local government executing only 63 percent of its health budget and central government executing 135 percent of its health budget.

For decentralization to work, matching of functions needs to be carefully considered. For example, transferring authority to hire and fire staff members may have less of an effect if authority on setting the skills mix is not transferred as well (that is, the local government might be able to select which individual to hire, but it could not select whether to hire a doctor or a nurse because of fixed staffing norms). Authority to set salaries might not be useful unless either (a) facilities have flexibility in how much of their budget can be used to pay health workers or (b) facility budgets are adjusted on the basis of local salary levels. In other words, an appropriate match needs to be made between fiscal and administrative functions.

Moreover, it is extremely important to consider to what level authority should be transferred down. Two factors are important. First, as noted, sufficient capacity to carry out key functions at that level is a must. Second, legal authority for the level to carry out those functions is also required. For example, if hiring authority is to be transferred down to the facility level, facilities need to be separate legal entities that employ staff. If hiring authority is transferred to the district level, then districts need to be legal entities separate from the central level.

Removing the Health Workforce from the Civil Service

Subject to certain conditions, health workers could be removed from the civil service and the overall wage bill so that the ministry of health has full control over both the size and the use of the health wage bill. This policy option is the most aggressive discussed here and requires significant public sector reform, with considerable risk (see box 1.1). Under this policy option, health workers are no longer direct civil service employees. They are employed directly either by facilities or by central, regional, or district agencies that have some degree of autonomy from the government (for example, boards of health in Zambia). Moreover, the health wage bill is no longer part of the overall wage bill. Health worker salaries are funded from block grants that cover all operating expenses. This policy option affects two main areas: (a) the size of the health wage bill and (b) how health wage bill resources are used.

The size of the health wage bill. This policy option enjoys two main advantages related to the size of the health wage bill. First, delinking the health sector from the civil service makes resources more fungible because the budgeting process for the health wage bill and for nonwage bill items would no longer be disconnected. Therefore, within a given health budget (that is, the block grant), facilities or agencies that employ health workers would have more control over how the budget (the block grant) is allocated across wage and nonwage items. The facility would have flexibility in combining the various inputs in the most effective way for delivering quality services. Second, if the government wishes to increase health spending significantly—either through domestic resources or with donor aid—but has a fiscal ceiling on the overall wage bill, the health workforce can expand without affecting the overall wage bill. The government would simply increase health spending through increased block grants. Facilities could then expand staffing levels. Because no part of the block grant is counted as part of the overall wage bill, increasing the grant would not affect the size of the overall wage bill.

Several challenges are associated with this policy option. First, the proper legal framework needs to be in place. Agencies or facilities need to have legal authority to employ health workers. This policy option may not be available in countries where agencies do not have such authority or where such a legal reform is not feasible.

Second, as the country studies demonstrate, either expansion of the overall wage bill may be limited by explicit wage bill ceilings (as in Kenya, for example) or the government may set a limit on the fiscal deficit (as in Rwanda, for example). In the latter case, the expansion of the overall wage bill is indirectly limited because it increases the overall deficit, all else being equal. This policy option is most appropriate in situations where an explicit wage bill ceiling exists, rather than an indirect one, because removing the health wage bill from the overall wage bill and including it in block grants reduces the overall wage bill but has no direct effect on the fiscal deficit.

Third, labor regulations need to be unrestrictive. When health workers are employed on contracts in public sector facilities, they are often subject to government labor laws, even if they are not civil servants. These labor laws may govern the terms of work, staffing norms, and types of contracts. One such stipulation of labor laws that might be of concern guarantees a permanent position in the civil service after a certain period of service under contract in the public sector. Such labor laws generate contingent liabilities for the government because hiring more health workers on contracts, in the long run, leads to more permanent employees in the civil service and increases in the overall wage bill. Two methods can be used to mitigate this contingent liability effect. The first is to change the labor laws so that workers do not automatically receive guaranteed permanent employment. The second is to make health facilities fully autonomous so that they are legally separate entities from the government even though they are funded through government resources. In this case, the government labor laws would not fully apply to these health facilities. Both of these mitigating effects would require further public sector reform.

Fourth, strong lines of accountability need to be in place. The ministry of health would have significant autonomy in setting the size of the health wage bill and terms of work—including salaries—for health workers under this policy option. Without strong accountability measures, this option could result in little improvement in health workforce performance and service delivery. In Zambia, the delinkage of the health boards from the Ministry of Health was fraught with irregularities. Health workers received more favorable terms of service, and the wage bill consumed an increasing share of the health budget, thereby restricting investment in important infrastructure. The health boards were ultimately abolished as a result.

Several mechanisms can be considered for ensuring accountability. An input-focused control mechanism could be used that sets an upper limit on the share of the block grant that could be used for the wage bill. Alternatively, an output-based control mechanism could be used, in which the facilities or agencies simply were held accountable for meeting service delivery targets and quality standards.

Rwanda provides a good example of how some of the implementation challenges associated with this policy option can be addressed. Recently, the health sector was partially removed from the overall wage bill. Salaries of health workers are still paid out of the overall wage bill, but performance-based allowances—which are a main source of remuneration and can be as large as 86 percent of basic salary—are paid out of block grants given to facilities and are not counted as part of the overall wage bill. The block grants can also be used to hire additional workers on contracts, but at the time of study this option was permitted only for support staff members, not clinical staff members. The allowances are paid in accordance with a well-defined formula, and the amount of the block grant that can be used for paying health workers is limited to 75 percent. No systematic evaluation of the reform has been done yet, but early indications suggest that the system has provided districts and facilities much more control over the health wage bill. Facilities can supplement the salary budget (which comes from earmarked central funds) and provide the necessary incentives to improve retention and health worker performance. The new system has also increased overall health worker wages—on a performance basis—without affecting the overall wage bill.

Use of wage bill resources. Taking the health workers out of the civil service has several advantages that relate to use of health wage bill resources. First, salary scales would no longer be bound by the overall civil service salary scale, and no need would exist to negotiate for separate allowances for the health sector, which is often politically difficult. More flexibility over remuneration policy can be beneficial because the incentives provided by the current salary and allowance structure for health workers in the public sector—both in the country case studies and in the literature review in appendix D—generally do not promote good health workforce performance. The performance-based allowance system implemented recently in Rwanda provides a good example: the health sector has taken advantage of increased autonomy over setting allowances to improve incentives for productivity and quality of care. Independent salary scales can also remove effects that altering health worker salaries can have on other sectors; such scales have been found to have a significant fiscal effect.

Second, the number of steps and the number of actors in the recruitment process would be drastically reduced. The health sector would not need to follow civil service recruitment procedures. The country case studies show that this requirement is a major administrative bottleneck preventing full execution of the health wage bill. In Kenya, the Ministry of Health was granted authority to bypass the centralized system and recruit staff members (within a certain wage bill budget), and it reduced recruitment times dramatically.

However, there are also major challenges (box 1.4). Sufficient capacity is necessary within the ministry of health to manage key human resources for health functions strategically with the right incentives and lines of accountability in place. In several of the country case studies, it is doubtful that this enabling condition is satisfied. In Zambia, when the boards of health were granted autonomy over recruitment, mostly administrative and support staff members were hired, not clinical workers. The increased autonomy over wage setting simply led to wage increases that were not linked to performance as well as to crowding out of important nonwage health expenditure, such as capital investments.

The case of Kenya demonstrates how important capacity building is when autonomy over recruitment and compensation practices is granted to the ministry of health. Through the Emergency Hiring Program, significant investments were made in capacity, including computerization of

Box 1.4

Political Economy of Removing Health Workers from the Civil Service

Where delinking the health workforce from the civil service has been tried, the results reveal the considerable difficulties in this process that stem from political economy factors. Delinkage caused concerns among health workers about job stability, security, and remuneration. The governance and accountability dimension of this policy reform clearly needs to be deeply considered before implementation begins. For instance, in both the Philippines and Zambia, health workers effectively halted the delinkage process even after implementation had begun. Their disgruntlement stemmed from uncertainty over whether their rights and remuneration levels would be maintained without the backing of the civil service administration. This opposition occurred despite the initial intent of the reform process to improve terms of service for health workers to address shortages and inequities.

The Philippines and Uganda, where the central governments attempted to delink the health workforce from the overall civil service, provide examples. The governments transferred all hiring and firing authority to local governments; however, because of political opposition by health workers, the central government maintained authority over salary levels, benefits, and terms of service. Although this partial transfer of authority was not the initial intent of the reform process in both countries, it allowed the government to effectively decentralize certain key human resource management functions in light of political concerns of health workers. After encountering implementation difficulties, the government found focusing on the delinkage of strategic areas of human resources for health management more politically and practically feasible, while maintaining the central civil service administration's control over the actual wage bill.

For delinkage to be effective, government health workers must be comfortable with the newly created purchaser-provider system. They must have assurance that their rights will not be reduced from the levels they previously had a regular civil servants because of a disparate relationship with the government terms of service. Furthermore, civil service reform of this magnitude will have to be accompanied by other coordinated policy measures to ensure successful implementation.

In many developing countries, the political and regulatory context will simply impede complete delinkage. Developed countries, in contrast, have effectively delinked government health workers. The introduction of the National Health

(continued)

Box 1.4 *(Continued)*

Service in the United Kingdom put into place a purchaser-provider health care system and effectively delinked health workers from the overall civil service. Many lessons emerge from the U.K. experience. First, although it slowed the reform process, legal provisions were put into place to protect employment rights and conditions of employment during the transition period, thus providing the necessary conditions to get buy-in from health worker unions. Second, delinkage of the health workforce occurred within the context of overall health sector reform and decentralization. This overhaul of the system changed incentives among local health managers and health workers, as well as provided more flexible arrangements for hiring, remuneration, and training. Delinking in the United Kingdom was successful because of well-thought-out and staged policy implementation, as well as an effective governance structure that had the confidence of health workers.

Sources: Bossert and Beauvais 2002; Buchan 2000; country case studies.

records and creation of a just-in-time database of vacancies that was driven in part by significant support from development partners. Short-term contracts were used, and the staff was monitored regularly. Retention was extremely high, and the program was a success. Because donor agencies funded the program, there was an additional line of accountability.

In the Dominican Republic, the Secretaría de Estado de Salud Pública y Asistencia Social (Ministry of Public Health and Social Assistance, or SESPAS), the main employer of health workers in the public sector, has a high degree of authority over compensation and terms of work. In response to union pressures to increase wages and a fiscal constraint on the health wage bill, SESPAS recently agreed to reduce the minimum hours worked in public facilities to 20 hours per week. Salaries remained unchanged. The implications for service delivery for the poor could be significant.

Given the numerous risks and extensive list of enabling conditions, the policy option of removing the health sector from the civil service and the overall wage bill is unlikely to be available in many developing countries. This policy option should be considered only if it is preceded or accompanied by the necessary legal and regulatory reforms; significant capacity building, including accurate data systems, managerial training, and monitoring of staff performance; and a proper incentive system for accountability of the ministry of health.

Notes

1. The overall wage bill includes salaries and most allowances paid to all employees of the government. The health wage bill comprises the salaries and most allowances of all health workers in the public sector.

2. For Kenya and Zambia, the years covered by the data in the scatter plot are different from the period discussed in the previous section. The period covered by the scatter plot is the expansionary period for the overall wage bill, whereas the discussion focuses on whether the health sector was prioritized during the period of overall wage bill cutbacks.

3. As a former minister of finance in Ghana stated recently in a keynote address at the Global Forum for Human Resources for Health—a high-level global conference organized by the Global Health Workforce Alliance: "We keep giving health more and more money for salaries; in the end what do we get?"

4. The 5.36 percent represents the original 2.70 percent to cover the health sector plus the 2.66 percent to cover the education sector.

5. What is "right" must be based on some objective measure, such as the types of health workers whose skills are best matched to the health care needs of the population.

6. An important example of this situation exists in Ghana, where an additional duty hours allowance was put in place to reward hours worked in excess of the standard workweek in the civil service. Staff members were to receive additional payment based on hours worked, with ceilings set for maximum hours. Initially, only doctors were eligible, but the allowance was later extended to nurses and other staff members. The allowance became a fixed salary top-up completely unrelated to performance and was abolished in 2007.

References

Action Aid International. 2004. *Blocking Progress: How the Fight against HIV/AIDS Is Being Undermined by the World Bank and International Monetary Fund.* Washington, DC: Action Aid International.

Ambrose, Soren. 2006. "Preserving Disorder: IMF Policies and Kenya's Health Care Crisis." Global Policy Forum, New York. http://www.globalpolicy.org/socecon/bwi-wto/imf/2006/0601imfhealth.htm.

Anand, Sudhir, and Till Bärnighausen. 2004. "Human Resources and Health Outcomes: Cross Country Econometric Study." *Lancet* 364 (9445): 1603–9.

Anderson, James, Gary Reid, and Randi Ryterman. 2003. "Understanding Public Sector Performance in Transition Countries: An Empirical Contribution." Poverty Reduction and Economic Management Unit, Europe and Central Asia Region, World Bank, Washington, DC. http://www1.worldbank.org/publicsector/civilservice/UPSP%20final.pdf.

Banteyerga, Hailom, Aklilu Kidanu, and Kate Stillman. 2006. *The Systemwide Effects of the Global Fund in Ethiopia: Final Study Report.* Bethesda, MD: Partners for Health Reform *plus* Project, Abt Associates.

Bossert, Thomas J., and Joel C. Beauvais. 2002. "Decentralization of Health Systems in Ghana, Zambia, Uganda, and the Philippines: A Comparative Analysis of Decision Space." *Health Policy and Planning* 17 (1): 14–31.

Buchan, James. 2000. "Health Sector Reform and Human Resources: Lessons from the United Kingdom." *Health Policy and Planning* 15 (3): 319–25.

Center for Global Development. 2007. *Does the IMF Constrain Health Spending in Poor Countries? Evidence and an Agenda for Action.* Washington, DC: Center for Global Development. http://www.cgdev.org/doc/IMF/IMF_Report.pdf.

Chaudhury, Nazmul, and Jeffrey S. Hammer. 2004. "Ghost Doctors: Absenteeism in Rural Bangladeshi Health Facilities." *World Bank Economic Review* 18 (3): 423–41.

Das, Jishnu, and Paul J. Gertler. 2007. "Variations in Practice Quality in Five Low-Income Countries: A Conceptual Overview." *Health Affairs* 26 (3): 296–309.

Das, Jishnu, and Jeffrey S. Hammer. 2004. "Strained Mercy: The Quality of Medical Care in Delhi." Policy Research Working Paper 3228, World Bank, Washington, DC. http://ssrn.com/abstract=610269.

Dussault, Gilles, and Maria Cristina Franceschini. 2006. "Not Enough There, Too Many Here: Understanding Geographical Imbalances in the Distribution of the Health Workforce." *Human Resources for Health* 4: 12.

Dussault, Gilles, and Marko Vujicic. 2008. "The Demand and Supply of Human Resources for Health." In *International Encyclopedia of Public Health*, vol. 2, ed. Kris Heggenhougen and Stella Quah, 77–84. San Diego: Academic Press.

Fedelino, Annalisa, Gerd Schwartz, and Marijn Verhoeven. 2006. "Aid Scaling Up: Do Wage Bill Ceilings Stand in the Way?" IMF Working Paper 06/106, International Monetary Fund, Washington, DC. http://www.imf.org/external/pubs/ft/wp/2006/wp06106.pdf.

Ferrinho, Paulo, Wim Van Lerberghe, Inês Fronteira, Fátima Hipólita, and André Biscaia. 2004. "Dual Practice in the Health Sector: Review of the Evidence." *Human Resources for Health* 2: 14. http://www.human-resources-health.com/content/2/1/14.

Franco, Lynne Miller, Sara Bennett, and Ruth Kanfer. 2002. "Health Sector Reform and Public Sector Health Worker Motivation: A Conceptual Framework." *Social Science and Medicine* 54 (8): 1255–66.

Gottret, Pablo, and George Schieber. 2006. *Health Financing Revisited: A Practitioner's Guide.* Washington, DC: World Bank.

Gwatkin, Davidson R., Shea Rutstein, Kiersten Johnson, Eldaw Suliman, Adam Wagstaff, and Agbessi Amouzou. 2007. *Socio-economic Differences in Health, Nutrition, and Population within Developing Countries.* Washington, DC: World Bank.

Hongoro, Charles, and Charles Normand. 2006. "Health Workers: Building and Motivating the Workforce." In *Disease Control Priorities in Developing Countries,* ed. Dean T. Jamison, Joel G. Breman, Anthony R. Measham, George Alleyne, Mariam Claeson, David B. Evans, Prabhat Jha, Anne Mills, and Philip Musgrove, 1309–22. New York: Oxford University Press.

IMF (International Monetary Fund). 2007. "Zambia: 2007 Article IV Consultation—Staff Report; Staff Statement; Public Information Notice on the Executive Board Discussion; and Statement by the Executive Director for Zambia." IMF Country Report 08/41, IMF, Washington DC. http://www.imf.org/external/pubs/ft/scr/2008/cr0841.pdf.

Joint Learning Initiative. 2004. *Human Resources for Health: Overcoming the Crisis.* Cambridge, MA: Global Equity Initiative, Harvard University.

Kenya Ministry of Finance. 2007. "The Medium Term Budget Strategy Paper, 2007/08–2009/10." Kenya Ministry of Finance, Nairobi.

Klingner, Donald E., and John Nalbandian. 2002. *Public Personnel Management: Contexts and Strategies,* 445–98. New York: Pearson Education.

Kombe, Gilbert, David Galaty, Raj Gadhia, and Catherine Decker. 2005. *The Human and Financial Resource Requirements for Scaling Up HIV/AIDS Services in Ethiopia.* Bethesda, MD: Abt Associates.

Kurowski, Christoph, Kaspar Wyss, Salim Abdulla, and Anne Mills. 2007. "Scaling Up Priority Health Interventions in Tanzania: The Human Resources Challenge." *Health Policy and Planning* 22 (3): 113–27.

McCoy, David, Sara Bennett, Sophie Witter, Bob Pond, Brook Baker, Jeff Gow, Sudeep Chand, Tim Ensor, and Barbara McPake. 2008. "Salaries and Incomes of Health Workers in Sub-Saharan Africa." *Lancet* 371 (9613): 675–81.

OECD (Organisation for Economic Co-operation and Development). 2007. *International Migration Outlook 2007.* Paris: OECD.

Okuonzi, Sam Agatre. 2004. "Dying for Economic Growth? Evidence of a Flawed Economic Policy in Uganda." *Lancet* 364: 1632–37.

Ooms, Gorik, and Ted Schrecker. 2005. "Expenditure Ceilings, Multilateral Financial Institutions, and the Health of Poor Populations." *Lancet* 365 (9473): 1821–23.

Preker, Alexander S., Marko Vujicic, Yohana Dukhan, Caroline Ly, Hortenzia Beciu, and Peter Nicolas Materu. 2008. "Scaling Up Health Professional Education: Opportunities and Challenges for Africa." Paper prepared for the Task Force for Scaling Up Education and Training for Health Workers, Global Health Workforce Alliance, World Bank, Washington, DC.

Rauch, James E., and Peter B. Evans. 2000. "Bureaucratic Structure and Bureaucratic Performance in Less Developed Countries." *Journal of Public Economics* 75 (1): 49–71.

Recanatini, Francesca, Alessandro Prati, and Guido Tabellini. 2005. "Why Are Some Public Agencies Less Corrupt Than Others? Lessons for Institutional Reform from Survey Data." Paper presented at PREM Week Forum, World Bank, Washington, DC, October.

Reid, Gary J. 2005. "The Political Economy of Civil Service Reform in Albania." World Bank, Washington, DC.

Ruwoldt, Paul, and Philip Hassett. 2007. "Zanzibar Health Care Worker Productivity Study: Preliminary Study Findings." Capacity Project, IntraHealth International, Chapel Hill, NC. http://www.capacityproject.org/images/stories/files/zanzibar_productivity_study.pdf.

Serneels, Pieters, Magnus Lindelow, José G. Montalvo, and Abigail Barr. 2006. "For Public Service or Money: Understanding Geographical Imbalances in the Health Workforce." *Health Policy and Planning* 22 (3): 128–38.

Verhoeven, Marijn, and Alonso Segura. 2007. "IMF Trims Use of Wage Bill Ceilings." *IMF Survey Magazine*, September 5. http://www.imf.org/external/pubs/ft/survey/so/2007/POL095A.htm.

Vujicic, Marko. 2005. "Macroeconomic and Fiscal Issues in Scaling Up Human Resources for Health in Low-Income Countries." Background paper prepared for *The World Health Report 2006: Working Together for Health*. World Bank, Washington, DC. http://www.who.int/hrh/documents/macroeconomic_fiscal_issues.pdf.

Vujicic, Marko, Eddie Addai, and Samuel Bosomprah. 2006. "Methodology for Measuring the Productivity of the Health Workforce in Ghana." Ministry of Health, Accra.

Vujicic, Marko, and Robert Evans. 2005. "The Impact of Deficit Reduction on the Nursing Labor Market in Canada: Unintended Consequences of Fiscal Reform." *Applied Health Economics and Health Policy* 4 (2): 99–110.

Vujicic, Marko, and Pacal Zurn. 2006. "The Dynamics of the Health Labor Market." *International Journal of Health Planning and Management* 21 (2): 105–15.

Wagstaff, Adam, and Mariam Claeson. 2004. *The Millennium Development Goals for Health: Rising to the Challenges*. Washington, DC: World Bank.

WHO (World Health Organization). 2006. *World Health Report 2006: Working Together for Health*. Geneva: World Health Organization. http://www.who.int/whr/2006/en/index.html.

———. 2007. "Task Shifting to Tackle Health Worker Shortages." World Health Organization, Geneva, Switzerland. http://www.who.int/healthsystems/task_shifting_booklet.pdf.

Wood, Angela. 2006. "IMF Macroeconomic Policies and Health Sector Budgets." WEMOS Foundation, Amsterdam. http://www.wemos.nl/Documents/ wemos_synthesis_report_final.pdf.

World Bank. 2006. *Zambia Education Sector Public Expenditure Review.* Washington, DC: World Bank.

———. 2007. *World Development Indicators 2007.* Washington, DC: World Bank.

———. 2008. *Public Sector Reform: What Works and Why? An IEG Evaluation of World Bank Support.* Washington, DC: World Bank.

CHAPTER 2

Background Country Study for Kenya

"Kenya urgently needs to hire 10,000 additional professionals in the public health sector. We have to put our foot down and employ."

—Enock Kibunguchy, assistant minister for health, commenting on Kenya's health workforce crisis (Ambrose 2006)

The government of Kenya increasingly recognizes that human resource development is key to improved health service delivery and health sector transformation. The health sector is one of the central pillars of the Economic Recovery Strategy and a key pillar of Kenya Vision 2030. The National Health Sector Strategic Plan recognizes very explicitly that the availability of skilled workers in adequate numbers is critical for the realization of the sector mission to deliver quality and accessible health services (Kenya Ministry of Health 2005b). According to the government, the Kenyan health care system is weakened because of inadequate numbers of personnel in key areas of the health sector, inequitable distribution of health personnel, and attrition of highly trained health workers. The Ministry of Health has estimated that the health sector today requires 7,000 additional health workers to deliver essential services to the population (Kenya Ministry of Health 2007a).

The Health Wage Bill in Kenya

The budget for the health wage bill in the public sector is determined through a three-stage process. The government prepares a budget for the public sector wage bill covering all sectors. The Ministry of Health prepares an overall health sector budget that includes a line item for the health sector wage bill. Negotiations within the government determine the allocations of the total public sector wage bill budget to each sector, including health. Each of these processes is discussed. The process is summarized in table 2.1.

Budget for the Public Sector Wage Bill

Curtailing the public sector wage bill is important to avoid a crowding-out effect. Expanding the public sector wage bill can limit fiscal space for implementing poverty reduction programs. However, it is equally

Table 2.1   Main Steps in the Budget Cycle

Approximate timing	Step	Actors
September–November	Prepare Budget Outlook Paper.	Treasury and Macroeconomic Working Group
August–December	Conduct public expenditure review (including review of ministerial PER).	Treasury
December	Issue Medium-Term Expenditure Framework guidelines and Budget Outlook Paper.	Treasury
December	Issue revised budget circular.	Treasury
December	Submit district inputs to ministry headquarters.	Line ministries
January–February	Submit revised estimates.	Line ministries
February–April	Develop and submit budget strategy paper.	Treasury and Macroeconomic Working Group
February	Hold sector hearings.	Treasury and Ministry of Planning and National Development
April–May	Develop itemized budget.	Line ministries
End of May	Send budget estimates to cabinet.	Ministry of Finance
End of May	Estimates printed.	Treasury
June	Present budget to Parliament for approval.	Ministry of Finance
July	New financial year starts.	

Sources: Kenya Ministry of Finance 2007a; WEMOS Foundation 2005, annex 1.

important to strike a balance between macroeconomic targets and the need to increase the health budgets if Kenya is both to make health services accessible and to ensure that it achieves its Millennium Development Goals (MDGs).

Managing the size of the public sector wage bill is important, as it can cause macroeconomic volatility. High government wages and large employment can push up the wage bill and crowd out other spending. Government wage increases could feed into a general wage-price spiral that undermines competitiveness; they could also result in fiscal slippages (Fedelino, Schwartz, and Verhoeven 2006).

For several years, Kenya has had a large public sector wage bill relative to other countries in the region. As a percentage of gross domestic product (GDP), the public sector wage bill within Kenya was 8.0 percent in 2005 (figure 2.1). This figure is relatively high in comparison with that of other Sub-Saharan Africa countries. Figure 2.2 illustrates that Kenya's public sector wage bill is 36 percent of total government expenditure in 2005, also very high in relation to other Sub-Saharan African countries. The public sector wage bill in Kenya includes both salaries and fixed allowances (such as the housing allowance) but excludes pensions and reimbursable allowances for all government employees.[1]

In 2000, budget and wage ceilings were introduced along with the Medium-Term Expenditure Framework (MTEF) as part of the financial reforms initiated under the public sector reform program. Because the public expenditure trends were not consistent with the objectives of achieving sustained economic growth and poverty reduction, the MTEF approach was adopted to link policy making to planning and budgeting; to maintain fiscal discipline by establishing hard budget constraints; to facilitate expenditure prioritization across policies, programs, and projects; and to encourage better use of resources to achieve desired outcomes at the lowest level. The goal was to rationalize public expenditure and to improve the macroeconomic environment. The government policy was to reduce the overall expenditure in relation to GDP, thereby reducing the budget deficit (WEMOS Foundation 2005).

Actual targets for the public sector wage bill are set by the government on the advice of the Macroeconomic Working Group (MWG). The MWG comprises representatives from the Central Bank of Kenya, the Ministry of Finance, the Kenya Revenue Authority, and the Kenya Institute for Public Policy Research and Analysis. The targets are based on broad macroeconomic conditions and are often set without direct input from the various line ministries.

Figure 2.1 Public Sector Wage Bill as a Share of GDP, by Region, 2005

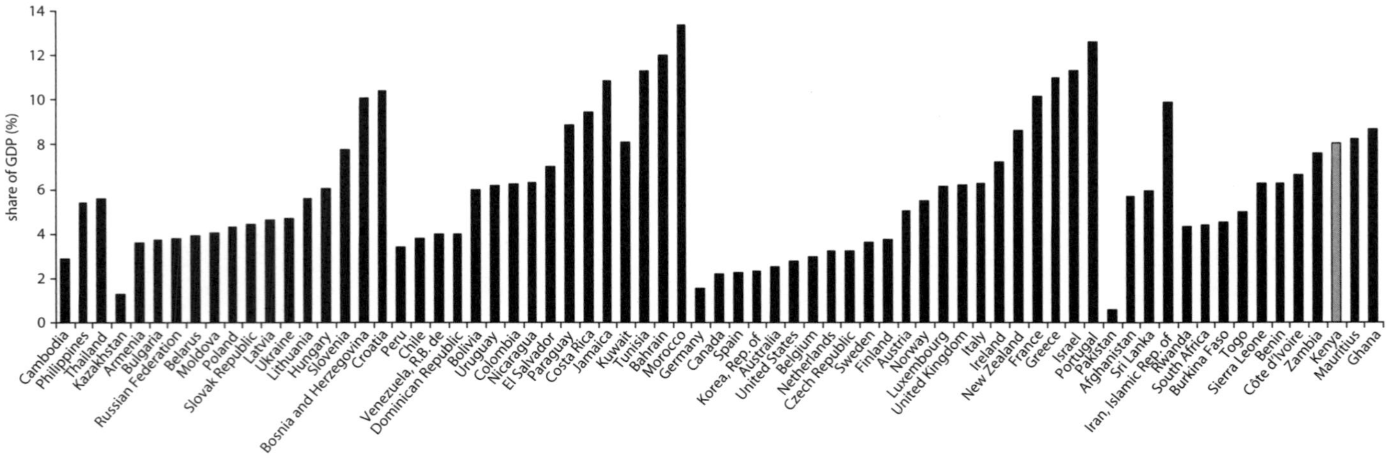

Share of GDP (%)

Cambodia
Philippines
Thailand
Kazakhstan
Armenia
Russian Federation
Bulgaria
Belarus
Moldova
Poland
Slovak Republic
Latvia
Ukraine
Lithuania
Hungary
Slovenia
Bosnia and Herzegovina
Croatia
Peru
Venezuela, R.B. de
Dominican Republic
Chile
Bolivia
Uruguay
Colombia
Nicaragua
El Salvador
Paraguay
Costa Rica
Jamaica
Kuwait
Tunisia
Bahrain
Morocco
Germany
Canada
Spain
Korea, Rep. of
United States
Australia
Belgium
Netherlands
Czech Republic
Sweden
Finland
Austria
Norway
Luxembourg
United Kingdom
Italy
Ireland
New Zealand
France
Greece
Portugal
Israel
Afghanistan
Pakistan
Iran, Islamic Rep. of
Sri Lanka
Rwanda
South Africa
Burkina Faso
Togo
Sierra Leone
Benin
Côte d'Ivoire
Zambia
Kenya
Mauritius
Ghana

Source: World Bank 2007.

Figure 2.2 Public Sector Wage Bill as a Share of Government Expenditure by Region, 2005

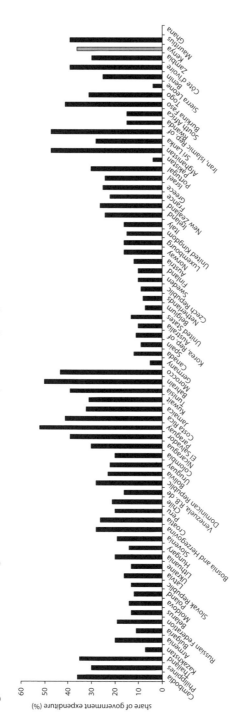

share of government expenditure (%)

Source: World Bank 2007.

Note: These numbers are based on World Bank data for total public sector compensation. Slight differences in the definition of *public sector compensation* can account for the small variation from government of Kenya data.

Historically, the International Monetary Fund (IMF) plays a significant role in setting the macroeconomic targets that in turn determine the national resource envelope. From 2003 to 2006, under the Poverty Reduction and Growth Facility (PRGF), the IMF included a wage bill ceiling as a condition of lending. The wage bill limits were necessary to contain a growing budget deficit and to ensure that resources were available for critical nonwage spending, including spending on medicines and school textbooks (Andrews 2007). Despite the ceiling, the government had plans to hire workers in the health sector. Subsequent reversal in policy was evident in the 2006/07 program, which was approved by the IMF Executive Board in April 2007, because that program did not include a limit on the wage bill. Despite increased hiring of teachers and health workers, the wage bill had declined to 7 percent of GDP (Andrews 2007).

The government has decided that the current wage bill level is too high, and recent budgets have included plans for large reductions. Figures 2.3 and 2.4 show the trends in the public sector wage bill. The wage bill peaked in 2003 at 9.2 percent of GDP (39 percent of government expenditure) and declined to 7.2 percent by 2007 (Kenya Ministry of Finance 2006). The government of Kenya has clearly made a concerted effort to reallocate resources away from wages and toward other expenditure categories. Both Treasury Circular 28/2004 and the MTEF guidelines for 2005/06 and 2007/08 instruct line ministries to base the wage bill budget on current authorized establishment. Any new recruitment will be allowed only following Treasury confirmation of availability of funding.

Figure 2.3   Public Sector Wage Bill as a Share of GDP, 2000–06

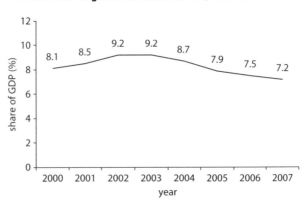

Sources: IMF 2003; Kenya Ministry of Finance 2007b.

Figure 2.4   Public Sector Wage Bill as a Share of Government Expenditure, 2000–07

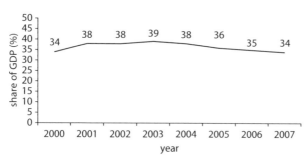

Sources: Kenya Ministry of Finance 2007a, table 3 figures; World Bank 2007.
Note: Figures for 2006 and 2007 are based on budget estimates.

Budget for the Health Sector Wage Bill

The budgeting of the health wage bill occurs in a multiple-stage process with input from both the Ministry of Finance and the Ministry of Health. The process begins with the government's Budget Outlook Paper, which is prepared by the MWG and outlines medium-term revenue and expenditure projections and provides preliminary sector ceilings for each ministry based on national priorities (WEMOS Foundation 2005). These ceilings are then used by sector working groups to allocate resources within a sector in the medium term. These sector budgets include a line item for the wage bill. However, budget preparation guidelines for line ministries often put strong restrictions on how much of the sector budget can be allocated to the wage bill. For example, in recent years, the guidelines have stated that the budget for the wage bill in each sector should be set on the basis of current staffing levels, and any incremental resources available for the total public sector wage bill will be allocated to sectors only later at the negotiations stage.[2]

Next, each ministry prepares a public expenditure review (PER). The PER has two purposes. First, it summarizes how the sector performed under the previous year's budget and what resources are required for the ministry to implement its sector strategy. Second, the PER shows the costing and resource requirements of the ministry, including the wage bill. These resource requirements take into account district department estimates of resource requirements. The PER stage is the opportunity for the ministries to provide input into the final budget results and is meant to create greater transparency and voice in the budgeting process (WEMOS Foundation 2005). One of the key aspects of the PER is an analysis of budget execution—the share of the previous year's budget that was actually spent. Underspending or overspending could be a sign of weak capacity in the ministry to carry out expenditures, represent poor planning and implementation of policies, or simply indicate that the ministry incurred some justifiable but unforeseen expenditures. The PER allows each sector to strengthen its rationale for additional wage bill resources. The current scenarios provided in the Ministry of Health's PER do not provide any strategic, costed content for human resources for health, including what would be done with incremental marginal wage bill resources and the expected benefits. There is much scope for improving the case for increased wage bill resources within the health sector.

Next, the central authority reviews the PERs and revises the sector expenditure ceilings in the budget strategy paper (BSP). The wage bill ceilings for each sector are also outlined in the BSP, and the rationale for prioritizing certain sectors is given.

The most recent BSP indicates that despite the aim to cut the public sector wage bill, the health sector remains a priority, and hiring will continue:

> Wage policy measures will include . . . flexibility to allow for recruitment of medical personnel in order to aim at reaching the optimum level of personnel for the health sector and to move toward achieving the MDGs. (Kenya Ministry of Finance 2007b: 23)

The BSP does not clearly outline whether the prioritization of the health sector will come at the expense of other sectors so that the overall public sector wage ceiling is met. Nor does it say how additional hiring in the health sector will be funded. Soon after the release of a BSP, public hearings are held so that all stakeholders can engage in a debate of the paper and propose amendments that they deem necessary before it is released to the cabinet. These views are consolidated, and the BSP is printed and released to the cabinet for discussion and approval (WEMOS Foundation 2005).

Each ministry must then prepare a budget in accordance with its sector strategy and the expenditure ceilings outlined in the BSP. Once all sector budgets are consolidated, they are presented to the cabinet for debate, and final budget ceilings are determined.

After the cabinet approves the government budget, a secondary process occurs that allows for supplemental funds to be allocated to ministries to fund new services, to cover any underprovisions, or to apply any realized savings on other services within the mandate of the ministry. In practice, supplementary budgets are presented to the Parliament of Kenya in

May, and the health sector has routinely used this process to supplement its budget (WEMOS Foundation 2005). For example, the Ministry of Health is responsible for staffing various health initiatives (such as Constituency Development Fund facilities[3]) that were put in place to service rural and local regions of the country, often without the assurance of the necessary allocation of additional resources. Supplementary budgets could be one way of obtaining additional funds for these mandates as well as covering costs that have not been properly planned for. For example, in January 2007, it was calculated that an extra KSh 1.2 billion would be required to cover a combination of a shortfall in wages, additional recruitment (for staffing of Constituency Development Fund facilities), and voluntary early retirement. An estimated further KSh 500 million would be required to cover a backlog of promotions that was to be cleared but had not been covered by the budget.

As a result of the budgeting process, the Ministry of Health has very limited control over how the budget for the health wage bill is set. The health wage bill is largely determined by historical staffing levels plus whatever increments are added during the budget negotiation stage. This situation is a consequence of the health sector being part of a national civil service. One major implication is that unless the public sector wage bill increases significantly, the only way to scale up the health workforce in the public sector is for the government to reallocate wage bill resources away from other sectors. As noted earlier, hiring in the health sector is the government's stated priority.

In recent years, donors have provided substantial resources to be used to pay the salaries of health workers. These resources have enabled the Ministry of Health to substantially increase its annual recruitment. Beginning in 2006, donors worked with the ministry to develop the Emergency Hiring Program (EHP) to address staffing shortages in underserved areas. Under the EHP, the U.S. President's Emergency Plan for AIDS Relief (PEPFAR); the Global Fund to Fight AIDS, Tuberculosis, and Malaria (GFATM); and the Clinton Foundation provided resources to support the hiring of health workers on three-year contracts tied to specific geographic areas. This funding had a substantial effect on the fiscal space for hiring health workers. In 2006, the majority of new recruitment in the public sector was funded by donors, and only 17.1 percent of such recruitment used health wage bill resources from the government. Under the EHP, funds are provided to the government, and staff members are employed by the Ministry of Health. Salaries and allowances paid are the same as those of other health workers in the ministry. The only significant difference is that EHP staff members are employed on a short-term contract with a gratuity equivalent to 31 percent of basic salary per year in place of a pension.

Because staff members are hired on short-term contracts, the EHP has not created a contingent wage bill liability for the government. There is no formal binding agreement that health care workers hired under the EHP will be converted to permanent staff members at the end of their contracts. The government has indicated that it intends to have the necessary wage bill resources after three years to do so, and it is clear health workers expect as much. But no formal agreement or commitment exists. Essentially, the donors have enabled the expansion of the health workforce and have bought time for the government to raise the necessary wage bill resources through economic growth. Table 2.2 provides a comparison of recruitment procedures followed by the government of Kenya and the EHP.

Table 2.2   Comparison of Government of Kenya and Emergency Hiring Program Recruitment Procedures

Characteristic	Government of Kenya	Emergency Hiring Program
Remuneration	—	Same as government but with gratuity of 31% of basic salary per year in place of pension
Tenure	Permanent	3-year contract
Recruitment process	Through PSC	Delegated by PSC to Ministry of Health with technical support from the Capacity Project and Deloitte & Touche; tight control to ensure no interference in selection process
Recruitment conditions	—	Merit based for all who meet job criteria, except candidates currently employed by faith-based organizations
Deployment conditions	Recruited to public service, so can be deployed anywhere	Can be deployed only to designated districts selected by Ministry of Health on the basis of staff shortages
Length of funding	Unlimited	3 years
Funding channel	—	Salaries paid directly to employees (PEPFAR funds) or directly to government (Clinton Foundation, GFATM)
Monitoring and evaluation	None	Detailed monthly follow up to monitor numbers and location of staff members
Time to fill a position	Varies; in some cases, 10 months from advertisement to interview	Letters of appointments sent within 4 months of advertisement; first batch of staff members in post within 5 months after receiving a 2-week induction course; second batch within 8 months

Source: World Bank analysis.

Results of the Wage Bill Budgeting Process

From 2000 to 2004, health spending as a share of government spending fell significantly, decreasing from 9.0 percent in 2001 to 6.1 percent in 2004. Nevertheless, spending by the Ministry of Health increased from KSh 395 (US$5.05) per capita in 2000 to KSh 578 (US$7.48) per capita in 2004. The health expenditure reductions during this period were focused mainly on nonsalary expenditures. The share of health spending devoted to the wage bill increased from 48 percent to 52 percent (figure 2.5). This increase suggests either a deliberate decision within the health sector to minimize staffing reductions or little flexibility to reduce staffing levels in the ministry because of the nature of employment in the public sector.

The health sector has accounted for a steadily increasing share of the public sector wage bill, indicating that the cutbacks in the public sector wage bill during 2001 to 2004 were much less severe for the health sector than for other sectors and that health was, indeed, prioritized in terms of public sector wage bill expenditure. The health sector accounted for 7.7 percent of the public sector wage bill in 2000 and 9.4 percent in 2004 (figure 2.6).

Health spending as a share of government spending is budgeted to increase significantly. According to the government budget, health spending by 2009 will account for 11 percent of government spending, thus reversing the previous downward trend. This plan shows a clear prioritization of health in the government budget (figure 2.5).

Figure 2.5   Health Expenditure as a Share of Government Expenditure and Health Wage Bill as a Share of Health Expenditure, 2000–09

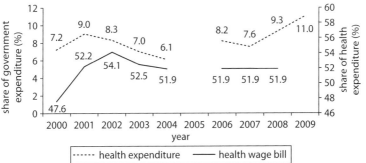

Sources: Kenya Ministry of Finance 2007b; Kenya Ministry of Health 2007b.

Note: Figures for 2006 through 2009 are based on budget estimates.

Figure 2.6   Health Wage Bill as a Share of Public Sector Wage Bill, 2000–07

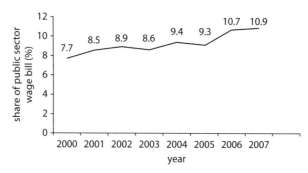

Sources: Kenya Ministry of Finance 2007b; Kenya Ministry of Health 2007b.

Note: Figures for 2006 and 2007 are based on budget estimates.

In the current Ministry of Health budget, the share of health spending devoted to the wage bill is set constant at 51.9% the current level. Hence, there appears to be very little strategic planning in the ministry when it comes to budgeting for the health wage bill. However, this lack of planning is understandable. Given that under the current budgeting process the ministry does not actually have much control over the health wage bill, budgeting for such expenditure in any strategic way may not make sense. Hence, future health wage bill amounts are simply set at their current level in the ministry's budget. If the ministry did have more control over the health wage bill, then it might outline year-by-year actions related to staffing that could be the basis for future wage bill budgets.

If the share of health spending devoted to the wage bill remains constant, as outlined in the Ministry of Health's budget, the health sector will continue to account for more and more of the public sector wage bill. Thus, further reallocations from other sectors will be necessary. Because of the ministry's projected increasing share of total government expenditure and the projection that the health wage bill will remain at a constant share of this budget, the health sector will account for 10.9 percent of the public sector wage bill in 2007 (figure 2.6). This increasing trend would suggest a prioritization of the health sector within the public sector wage bill. It is important to note that the government does not provide any sector-specific wage bill budgets beyond the current year. Thus, the information in figure 2.6 is not found in any budget documents and is simply constructed from the Ministry of

Health budget and the budget for the public sector wage bill. As noted earlier, the allocation of additional resources in the public sector wage bill to specific sectors is done on an annual basis, and there is no multiyear budgeting.

Budget execution of recurrent expenditures, including salaries, is very high in the Ministry of Health. The ratio of wages and salaries approved to actual wages and salaries is very close to 100 percent (table 2.3). This level is similar to budget execution levels for recurrent health spending in general. However, some indication exists that not all budgeted positions are filled. According to the most recent data from the Ministry of Health, there are currently 1,800 funded posts in the health sector (equivalent to 4.7 percent of the current workforce) for which budget has been approved and authority to hire granted but that are not filled (Kenya Ministry of Health 2007a). Possibly these positions were approved only in the most recent budget cycle, so the data do not take account of these positions.

Staffing levels in the health sector have increased steadily since 1998, including during the period of public sector wage bill reduction. This finding is consistent with an overall prioritization of the health sector within the public sector wage bill. Figure 2.7 shows the trend in hiring of new staff members by the Ministry of Health and the attrition level. There is clearly no downward trend in hiring, with a large increase in 2006. Attrition data were not available before 2004. It appears that during the cutbacks in the public sector wage bill, hiring continued in the ministry to a degree that led to an increasing level of health personnel in the country. The health sector seems to have been effectively shielded from the overall civil service reductions by increasing the share of the public sector wage bill devoted to health. This strategy allowed for a relatively stable level of recruitment of staff members. The large increase in recruitment levels in 2006 is mainly attributable to the donor-supported Emergency Hiring Program.

Table 2.3   Ministry of Health Budget Execution Rates, 2001/02–2004/05

Economic categories	Actual execution rates as a percentage of approved expenditure (%)			
	2001/02	*2002/03*	*2003/04*	*2004/05*
Total recurrent expenditure	100	100	104	101
Wages and salaries	103	100	101	99

Source: Kenya Ministry of Health 2007b.

Figure 2.7   Ministry of Health Staff Recruited and Lost, 2001–06

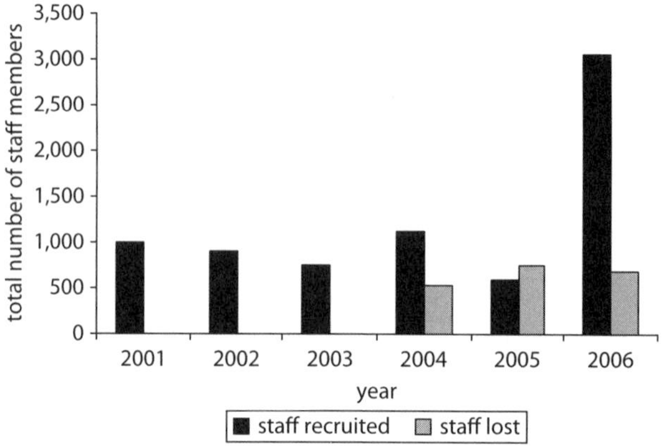

Source: Kenya Ministry of Health 2007b.

Unemployment among qualified health workers is significant, though the size of this pool can only be guessed. As part of the EHP hiring process, some useful information relating to the labor market was collected. Of the 4,466 suitably qualified applicants for the EHP, 2,064 (46 percent) were unemployed; 71 percent of these applicants were under the age of 30. This finding suggests that such applicants may never have been fully employed since graduation. Another example relates to medical interns. In 2006, of the 385 medical interns, a budget was provided for the recruitment of only 160. The remaining 225 eventually found jobs that were, in fact, not budgeted for in the public service.[4] These examples indicate that currently, unlike the situation in many countries in Sub-Saharan Africa, the labor market for health professionals in Kenya is quite loose.

Public Sector Employment of Health Workers

Within a given wage bill envelope, it is important to identify areas where the Ministry of Health can improve the efficiency of how wage bill resources are spent. Because the health sector is part of the national civil service, the health wage bill will always be constrained by the size of the public sector wage bill. In the future, the health sector must make the best use of existing resources. This section describes how health workers are currently recruited, deployed, and managed in the public sector.

Creating Funded Posts in the Health Sector

The creation of funded positions in the health sector does not rest with the Ministry of Health. As is the practice in the civil service in Kenya, such responsibilities ultimately lie with other agencies of the central government that are mandated to oversee personnel issues in the government. The Ministry of Health is responsible for developing staffing requirements for the health sector. Currently, these requirements are based on a workload assessment for implementing the Kenya Essential Package of Health (Kenya Ministry of Health 2006b). The Department of Personnel Management (DPM) of the Cabinet Office is responsible for maintaining a list of approved (but not necessarily funded) posts for each line ministry. This list is known as the "establishment," and it represents the overall staffing levels that have been approved (but not necessarily funded) for each line ministry. The current authorized establishment is 42,154. Health workers in the public sector in Kenya are part of a national civil service, so there is a single national establishment. As noted in the previous section, each year, through the budgeting process, the government allocates additional resources for the public sector wage bill to different ministries. The additional resources received by the Ministry of Health will be used to fund additional posts in the establishment, as well as to finance promotions and salary increases. Currently, 37,868 funded posts are filled, and an additional 1,800 funded posts have not been filled.

Thus, there are three steps to creating a funded vacancy in the health sector. First, the Ministry of Health submits a request to the DPM. Second, the DPM checks that the post is in the establishment for the health sector. Third, the DPM checks with the Treasury that sufficient resources from the public sector wage bill have been allocated to the health sector to fund the post. Then the DPM approves the position. A more detailed flowchart of the process of creating and filling a post is given in figure 2.8.

Recruiting Health Workers in the Public Sector

Recruitment of health workers into funded posts is managed centrally, with significant involvement of agencies outside of the Ministry of Health. Once the Ministry of Health gets approval that a post is funded and can be filled, it asks the Public Service Commission (PSC) to recruit for the position.[5] The first step is for the PSC to check the post against the relevant "schemes of service" to identify the qualifications needed for the position. The position is typically advertised in the newspaper as well as on the PSC Web site.

Figure 2.8   Flowchart of Process of Filling a Vacant Post

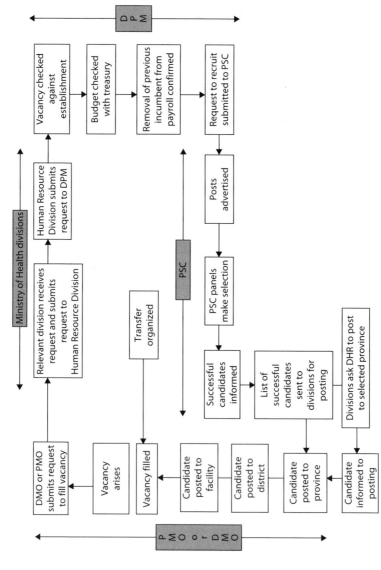

Source: Authors' representation.

Note: DMO = district medical officer; DPM = Department of Personnel Management; PMO = provincial medical officer; PSC = Public Service Commission.

Job advertisements do not typically specify the geographic location or type of facility where the post is located. Therefore, candidates presumably apply not knowing where they will be deployed and thus must be willing to accept deployment to any location in the country. Therefore, although it could be assumed that this system allows for efficient allocation of employees to areas of highest need, this process makes it very difficult to match individuals who are more willing to live in—and who are, thus, more likely to be retained in—remote areas to job vacancies in those areas.

Applicants are given 14 to 28 days to respond to the advertisement. The PSC then sorts the applications against the posts applied for and screens the applications for required qualifications to produce a "long list." A panel is then convened, consisting of experts from the relevant ministry, human resource experts from the PSC, and a commissioner, to draw up the short list.

Interviews for positions in the Ministry of Health are all held in Nairobi, with interviewees bearing the travel costs. In contrast, the Ministry of Education carries out its interviews locally. Having interviews in Nairobi poses a considerable burden on applicants from remote areas—the ones who are most likely to be willing to work in areas where vacancies are hard to fill. It also limits the rate at which candidates can be processed for job postings.

The current process of recruiting health workers into funded posts creates long delays. The target for processing time from when the Ministry of Health submits a request to the DPM to the when a successful candidate is selected is six months for a newly recruited staff member, and this time frame is included in the PSC's corporate performance contract. However, the current process takes much longer. About 1,200 health sector jobs were advertised in May 2006 by the PSC, but by January 2007, the interviews for a number of staff groups had yet to be conducted, according to the PSC. Interviews of 298 candidates for 51 Nursing Officer III posts were scheduled for mid-February 2007, about 10 months after the initial advertisement. However, one informant indicated that by April these interviews had still not taken place. One explanation for the delay was that in the interim the government had created a new Ministry of Youth Affairs to coincide with the Third Global Youth Employment Summit, which was held in Nairobi in September 2006. The new ministry needed to be staffed as a matter of priority. The cause of other delays is unclear, but the capacity of the PSC is certainly one important factor. The agency is made up of 8 officers responsible for screening, 10 clerical officers for filing and sorting, and 20 secretaries. The PSC is responsible for recruitment for the entire civil service—around 190,000 employees. Lack of capacity within the PSC presents an obvious bottleneck in the recruitment process.

Large efficiency gains are possible in the time it takes to fill funded posts. A recruitment initiative managed by the Capacity Project was launched in May 2006 under the donor-supported Emergency Hiring Program. This recruitment process was carried out using recruitment procedures that were similar to those of government. But the process was computerized, and recruitment authority was delegated by the PSC to the Ministry of Health's Department of Human Resources. It took only 10 days to create a short list of 2,600 health staff from a total of 7,000 applicants. The first successful recruits were in their posts by September 2007—less than five months after the jobs were advertised. The PSC is now developing an online job application facility. Applicants can currently find out online whether they have been selected for interviews and, eventually, whether they are successful in getting appointed.

There are indications that health care workers perceive corruption in the process of selecting candidates for employment. As mentioned earlier, the staff of the PSC is responsible for screening applicants for required qualifications to produce the long list, and a panel of experts from the Ministry of Health, human resource experts from the PSC, and a commissioner is responsible for drawing up the short list. In field visits conducted as part of this study, many health workers were surprisingly ready to discuss corruption in this process. A high-profile anticorruption drive is currently being implemented in Kenya. Calendars with anticorruption cartoons are a feature of many offices visited in the Ministry of Health. A survey of health sector staffing carried out in 2003 showed that political patronage had the biggest influence on the staff selection process, followed by nepotism and bribery, which shared the second position (Odundo and Wachira 2004). Some of the interviews clearly indicate that this pressure to influence recruitment and selection, as well as deployment, is still in place.

The Emergency Hiring Program has been extremely effective in increasing the transparency of the recruitment process. Because of corruption concerns, controls were put in place to prevent any tampering with the selection data. Invitations for interviews were posted in the newspaper to ensure that the correct candidates came. Concerns were also expressed about recruiting staff members from existing employers—in particular from the faith-based organizations, which pay slightly less than the government. In the end, the government did not include any special wording in the advertisements, and some recruitment did occur. Nevertheless, the majority of employees were recruited from the ranks of the unemployed (table 2.4).

Once hired, staff members are assigned by the Ministry of Health to provincial and district offices, which then assign them to facilities. This process does not appear to be strategic. The basis for assigning staff members is unclear, and again health workers perceive that this process is not transparent. Decisions both for deploying new entries and for moving individuals already in the system depend on accurate and up-to-date information on staffing at the different service levels, on workload, on vacancies, and on service delivery needs. The different technical departments collect information on services on a monthly basis, but it is unclear what information is collected on human resources for health. It is unclear what information is available to inform deployment decisions. Facilities may wait a year to have a vacancy filled. Decisions on deployment are referred to the relevant technical department that has information on service needs. For example, deployment of a nurse will be referred to the Nursing Department. The personal preferences of the individual also influence deployment. Some of those posted refuse to go to the post or attempt to negotiate a new posting that is closer to the center for training and other opportunities or closer to an urban area, where a private practice might be possible or a higher housing allowance might be received (Kenya Ministry of Health 2006a).

The transfer policies in the Ministry of Health are not conducive to addressing geographic imbalances. Following the initial deployment of employees, the ministry's policy states that staff members may be transferred to other locations for a number of different reasons. These reasons include promotions and staff requests to be transferred to more favorable locations. It is not clear whether ministry policies address other reasons

Table 2.4   Distribution of Short-Listed Candidates under Emergency Hiring Program, May 2006

Current status	Number of candidates
Unemployed	2,064
Privately employed	1,110
Other	661
Employed by faith-based organization	465
Employed by Ministry of Health	166
Employed by nongovernmental organization	0
Total	4,466

Source: Emergency Hiring Program statistics, Kenya Ministry of Health.

for reallocating staff, such as to implement strategic deployment or to address geographic imbalances. The ministry has a policy of not allowing staff members to stay in the same post for more than three years. This policy is not followed. Information collected on the length of time employees have been in their current stations indicates that 48.5 percent have stayed in their current working stations for more than five years. Hence, 60.6 percent of the employees should be transferred to new stations. According to the ministry, overstaying of some officers in the facilities has affected their performance in service delivery. Most affected are public health officers (Kenya Ministry of Health 2005a).

As shown in table 2.5, current deployment strategies have not resulted in an equitable distribution of staff—particularly for doctors and nurses. Nairobi (including Kenyatta National Hospital) and Central and Coast provinces are better staffed with doctors than the other provinces are. In Western and Nyanza provinces, there are 2 public sector doctors for every 100,000 people. In North Eastern province, the ratio is much worse, with 1 public sector doctor for 100,000 people. North Eastern province has 28 public sector nurses per 100,000 people; in contrast, Central province has 73 nurses for every 100,000 people. Interestingly, Nairobi has among the lowest level of staffing when it comes to nurses, with just 34 nurses for every 100,000 people. There are only 6 public sector clinical officers for every 100,000 people living in North Eastern province, 7 clinical officers for every 100,000 people in Central province, and 7 clinical officers for

Table 2.5   Selected Ministry of Health Cadres and Facility Distribution by Province, 2004

Provinces	Population (millions)	Number of facilities	Doctors per 100,000 population	Clinical officers per 100,000 population	Nurses per 100,000 population
Rift Valley	8,000,000	710	3	8	49
Eastern	5,100,000	418	3	6	55
Nyanza	4,800,000	291	2	6	40
Central	3,900,000	277	4	7	73
Western	3,900,000	164	2	5	45
Coast	2,800,000	204	4	7	50
Nairobi[a]	1,300,000	29	6	5	34
North Eastern	1,200,000	65	1	6	28

Source: Kenya Ministry of Health 2005a.
a. If Kenyatta National Hospital were included, the staffing ratio would be higher.

every 100,000 people in Coast province. This situation can likely be attributed to the way posts are allocated, the way staff members are deployed, and the fact that capacity to monitor whether health workers are actually working in their assigned locations is fairly weak.

Terms of Work in the Public Sector

The terms of work for health workers in the public sector are governed by Kenya's Code of Regulations (May 2006) for members of the civil service staff and by Ministry of Health policy. This section discusses tenure, remuneration, and promotion in the public sector.

Tenure. Appointments within the public service fall within the following main categories:

- Permanent and pensionable (lifetime)
- Permanent and nonpensionable (lifetime)
- Temporary (3–12 months, without gratuity)
- Casual (up to 3 months)
- Contract (for specific projects or for retirees, with gratuity)

Most employees in the Ministry of Health are on permanent and pensionable contracts. The hiring of health workers on short-term contracts is a fairly recent practice in Kenya, with only 2.3 percent of staff members on short-term or temporary contracts (table 2.6). In fact, until only recently, graduates of health-related basic training courses were guaranteed jobs in the public service. One key informant said that following a health worker strike in 2005, the government used the opportunity to hire temporary replacement personnel on contract. This idea of hiring on nonpermanent contracts has been taken forward with funding from several donors under the EHP, which is described in more detail later. Interestingly, 47 percent of permanent staff members in the Ministry of Health do not have a letter of confirmation verifying their position in the ministry, as required by ministry regulations (Kenya Ministry of Health 2005a).

The use of short-term contracts has increased considerably through the Emergency Hiring Program. Beginning in 2006, the government entered into an agreement to use funds from the Clinton Foundation, PEPFAR, and GFATM to hire more health professionals. Under the EHP, the employment contracts are linked to specific facilities. Applicants were drawn from all over Kenya, and because positions were advertised locally, it was possible to recruit candidates who were more likely to remain in

Table 2.6   Distribution of Ministry of Health Staff by Type of Contract, 2005

Facility type	Contract	Permanent and pensionable	Permanent without pension	Probation	Temporary	Total
Headquarters or division	6	1,207	134	94	31	1,472
Provincial medical office, Ministry of Health	2	1,123	83	111	113	1,432
Provincial hospital	13	3,349	305	268	145	4,080
District hospital	12	14,415	1,689	1,649	354	18,119
Health centers	2	3,776	595	466	51	4,890
Dispensaries	4	3,526	575	392	56	4,553
Specialized hospitals	2	516	102	36	9	665
Rural health training and demonstration centers	0	341	63	20	8	432
Total	41	28,253	3,546	3,036	767	35,643
Percentage of total	0.1	79.3	9.9	8.5	2.2	100

Source: Kenya Ministry of Health 2005a.

the job after being recruited. The use of short-term contracts was mainly a result of the short-term nature of the donor resources that supported the EHP. Interestingly, the program managed to effectively recruit health workers into underserved areas, with the most underserved areas receiving the most staff members (table 2.7). Only 1 percent of the candidates were posted in Nairobi.

Remuneration. Staff employed in government facilities can be divided into two categories: (a) those on the Ministry of Health payroll and (b) casual workers funded out of revenue generated by the facilities. One of the ways that managers compensate for the lack of available central funding for staff and effectively circumvent the personnel emolument ceilings is to use income generated from fees as a substitute. This income has been reduced with the changed policy on charging fees. There is a danger that facilities will have even greater staffing problems or that they will start using some of the operations budget to pay salaries.

Table 2.7   Emergency Hiring Program Statistics, 2006

Location of residence	Total applicants	Total qualified applicants (shortlisted)	Total selected applicants (deployed by Ministry of Health)
Nairobi	494	338	7
Central	1,197	898	71
Coast	224	143	49
Eastern	1,138	834	36
North Eastern	100	72	110
Nyanza	1,050	441	98
Rift Valley	1,674	1,247	149
Western	689	493	99
All locations	6,566	4,466	619

Source: Emergency Hiring Program statistics, Kenya Ministry of Health.

Casual workers are usually support staff members, such as cooks, cleaners, and security guards, though professional staff members can be employed as casual workers if sufficient funds are available. Off-budget casual contracting allows facility managers to deal with the constraints on hiring using government health wage bill funds. In some facilities, the proportion of casual workers may be quite high. In one provincial hospital, 15 percent of the total complement of 267 employees were employed on casual contracts (Kenya Ministry of Finance 2007b).

Staff members on the government payroll are placed according to job and grade on a single pay scale that is used across the public service. The scale ranges from "A" for the lowest cadre of staff, to "U," the level of the permanent secretary, who is the top civil service official in the respective ministry (table 2.8). Within each alphabetical grade, there are steps, which reflect the length of time and seniority within the respective pay grade. Pay is usually determined by the grade and step within the grade. The government publishes and regularly updates the pay scales.

Salary reviews in fiscal years 2004/05 and 2005/06 raised the average take-home pay for senior managers in the public service (job groups P–S) by 200 to 300 percent. The middle-level managers (job groups K–N) on the average received a 100 percent increase during the same period, while support staff members (job groups A–J) received on the average a 70 percent increase. These increments have been designed to decompress the pay scales as well as to offer competitive remuneration to the managerial and technical cadres. Whereas as of January 1, 2006, the medium-term target pay for senior managers had been met, the target pay had not been achieved for the lower cadres, which still

Table 2.8   Grades of a Sample of Categories of Health Worker

Category	Grade
Permanent secretary	U
Chief economist or statistician	R
Deputy chief financial officer	Q
Medical intern, medical officer, senior medical officer, or assistant director specialist	L–P
Chief nursing officer	Q
Deputy chief nursing officer	N
Assistant chief nursing officer	M
Senior enrolled nurse	K
Nursing officer I, II, or III	H–K
Enrolled nurse I, II, or III	G–J
Ungraded nurse I, II, or III	D–F
Laboratory technician	C–E
Support staff member	A–E

Source: Kenya Ministry of Health 2006a, annex 1.

required at least KSh 6.3 billion for salary increases during the next MTEF (Bor 2006).

Allowances make up a significant proportion of the overall earnings of government workers. One informant said that there were up to 87 different allowances. All allowances combined account for 45 percent of the total wage costs in the Ministry of Health. By far, the largest allowance is for housing; this allowance makes up, on average, 21 percent of total wage costs, as shown in table 2.9. However, on an individual employee basis, the housing allowance may be as high as 30 percent of the individual's total remuneration package. One respondent reported that the ministry is currently negotiating for an increase in the allowance for uniforms—apparently to act as a salary supplement.

The housing allowance is a strong incentive for resisting a transfer out of Nairobi. The allowance is provided to all government employees, according to their location within Kenya, and the allowance for Nairobi is the highest. The loss of a Nairobi housing allowance is considered a significant disincentive to accepting a transfer elsewhere. This situation implies that the allowance is not fully used for accommodation; instead, it acts as a salary top-up, either because people prefer to live in substandard accommodation or because it has been set at an artificially high rate.[6] A human resource mapping study states that 11,129 employees (or 31.2 percent of the staff surveyed) are drawing a higher housing allowance than that to which they are entitled, which raises important

Table 2.9   Monthly Salary and Allowance Type as a Percentage of Wage Costs in Health Ministry, 2004

Payment type	Amount (KSh)	Percentage of wage costs
Salaries	405,515,570	54.8
Housing allowance	156,517,476	21.1
Risk allowance	93,271,752	12.6
Nonpracticing allowance	33,118,142	4.5
Medical allowance	32,801,895	4.4
Extraneous	11,731,986	1.6
Hardship allowance	5,835,656	0.8
Transportation allowance	1,477,167	0.2
Administrative allowance	130,400	0.0
Special duty allowance	109,094	0.0
Acting allowance	2,735	0.0
Total	740,511,873	100

Source: Kenya Ministry of Health 2005a.

questions about how well the allocation of allowances is implemented (Kenya Ministry of Health 2005a).

Hardship allowances are provided to attract personnel to rural or hardship areas, but these allowances are small relative to overall compensation. They are unlikely to be adequate as a financial incentive for staff members to move to these areas. The allowance is just US$8 per month for a junior nurse and US$16 for more senior employees, which explains why the hardship allowance makes up only 1 percent of the overall remuneration costs in table 2.9. In contrast, teachers receive a hardship allowance equal to 30 percent of their salaries. Of Kenya's 71 districts, 22 are classified as hardship areas.

As an additional retention strategy, private practice is allowed in hardship areas. However, the prospects for additional income from a second job in the private sector tend to be much smaller in hardship areas than in urban centers.[7] In addition, there is evidence that private practice occurs even in urban setting, contrary to what is specified in the policy.[8] Recently, provisions have been made for people working in hardship areas to take two annual leaves instead of one as an additional incentive.

There is leakage in the implementation of both the housing allowance and the hardship allowance, but the government is making great advances in addressing this issue. An allowance follows the person, not the position. The additional cost of housing allowances received by staff members to which they were not entitled was calculated as KSh 12,296,600 per

Table 2.10   Entitled and Actual Housing Allowance Amounts, 2005

Region	Number of employees	Entitled housing allowance (KSh)	Actual housing allowance (KSh)	Variance (KSh)
Central	2,594	9,674,600	12,581,300	2,906,700
Coast	272	1,107,300	1,557,300	450,000
Nairobi	230	1,645,100	2,395,600	750,500
Grand total	11,129	38,487,000	50,783,600	12,296,600

Source: Kenya Ministry of Health 2005a.

month in 2005, accounting for about 2 percent of the overall wage costs of staff members covered by the study (table 2.10). For the hardship allowance, of the 35,643 staff members covered by the mapping, a small proportion (618, or less than 2 percent) were getting hardship allowances that they were not entitled to. It is calculated that this figure amounts to an overpayment of KSh 603,044 per month, or just under 1 percent of the overall wage costs of staff members covered by the study (Kenya Ministry of Health 2005a). From the statistics on the housing allowance, it is evident that a large number of health personnel are getting allowances to which they are not entitled. If the estimated KSh 155 million paid as wastage for housing and hardship allowances were instead used for recruitment of nurses and doctors, that amount could pay an additional 200 doctors or 600 nurses per year at the current salary scales (Kenya Ministry of Health 2005a). The government is putting measures in place to address the issue.

Promotion. Promotion possibilities are set out in the Schemes of Service, which indicate the minimum qualifications and experience required for career advancement. Promotion at lower grades (for example, grades H–J) is supposed to be automatic after three years. At higher levels (for example, grades K–L), the process becomes more competitive, given the limited number of higher-grade posts available.

Promotion is often delayed, and the process is perceived as lacking transparency, hence resulting in frustrations and low morale among health workers. In fact, the ministry currently has a backlog of promotions that should have occurred automatically but have not been made since 1996. This frustration at the lack of promotion is said to have a serious effect on staff morale. A recent survey suggests that these delays in some cases are deliberately used as a means of rent seeking by clerks at the ministry's headquarters (Odundo and Wachira 2004). Rent seeking, however, may not entirely account for the multiyear backlog in what should be a routine process.

Reforms to improve the process of promotion and good performance have been introduced, but rollout has been slow. The public sector reforms include strategies to improve performance using a results-based management initiative. Such strategies include the use of performance contracts, from the permanent secretary down to support staff members. This process is slowly being rolled out, but the rewards and sanctions have not been fully identified. Implementation seems to have been limited so far to the central-level ministry, as the few cases where performance contracts were issued were at the central level. No contracts have been identified at the provincial level and below. If properly implemented, this initiative has the potential to improve the general performance of the staff. For instance, the director of human resource management in the Ministry of Health, whose performance contract is set by the permanent secretary, said she had been given the target of recruiting 3,000 extra staff members by June 2007 through the emergency hiring process.

Key Messages

The government of Kenya's overall wage bill policy is one of several factors that have limited the scaling up of the health workforce. Given that the health sector is part of the national civil service, the budget for the health wage bill is largely beyond the direct control of the Ministry of Health. The health sector competes with other sectors for additional wage bill resources. The Ministry of Finance and ultimately the cabinet make the final decision on how additional wage bill resources in the current budget are to be allocated across sectors.

A ceiling was placed on the overall government wage bill between 2003 and 2006. This ceiling was, in fact, a condition of lending under the IMF's PRGF program. The government policy during this period was to insulate the health sector from the overall wage bill reductions and to prioritize hiring in the health sector. The evidence suggests that such a prioritization did in fact happen. Wage bill resources were reallocated to the health sector away from other sectors.

However, even with a prioritization of the health sector within the overall wage bill, the Ministry of Health was able to maintain hiring only at historic levels, which are not that far above what is needed simply to compensate for retirement, resignation, death, and migration. Scaling up the health workforce significantly, within the restrictive wage bill policy, was simply not possible.

In the future, the overall wage bill policy is likely to constrain the scaling up of the health workforce even more. According to recent data, 1,800 funded positions have not been filled in the health sector. In the very short term, therefore, increased funding for the health wage bill is not a major issue. However, once these positions are filled—and filling them will not be difficult given the large pool of unemployed health workers—the situation will be different.

Even though there is no overall wage bill ceiling in Kenya under the IMF's PRGF program, the government is clearly committed to reducing the size of the overall wage bill. Thus, the only way to expand hiring levels in the Ministry of Health in the medium to long term using domestic resources is to devote more and more of the overall wage bill to the health sector. However, recent experience suggests that even when such a change is made, it may be difficult to scale up hiring significantly.

Donor resources have been used successfully to scale up recruitment. Many of the negative consequences associated with using external resources to pay salaries have been avoided. Indeed, Kenya provides a good example of how donor resources have helped expand hiring in the heath sector dramatically. Beginning in 2006, donors worked with the Ministry of Health to develop the Emergency Hiring Program to address staffing shortages in underserved areas. Under this program, PEPFAR, GFATM, and the Clinton Foundation provided resources to support hiring of health workers on three-year contracts tied to specific geographic areas.

The EHP had a substantial effect on the fiscal space for hiring health workers in the public sector. In 2006, the majority of hiring in the health sector (83 percent) was funded by donors through the EHP. Under the EHP, funds are provided to the government, and staff members are employed by the ministry. Salaries and allowances are set at the same levels as those of other health workers in the ministry.

Because the staff members are hired on short-term contracts, there is no contingent wage bill liability created for the government. The government has indicated that it intends to have the necessary wage bill resources after three years to absorb the additional staff members, but there is no formal agreement of commitment. Essentially, the donors have bought time for the government to raise the necessary wage bill resources.

The Ministry of Health could be much more proactive in making the case for a higher share of overall wage bill resources. In fact, given the current restrictive policy on the overall wage bill, it must. There is considerable scope for the Ministry of Health to improve its strategy in negotiations with the

Ministry of Finance. The analysis of the budgeting process clearly shows that the ministerial PER is extremely important. The PER allows each sector to strengthen its rationale for additional wage bill resources. The current scenarios provided in the Ministry of Health's PER could provide more strategic, costed, incremental proposals for what additional wage bill resources would be used for, including the expected outcomes.

The budgeting process for wage bill and non-wage expenditure is not well coordinated. This lack of coordination leads to variations in wage and non-wage health expenditures that are unintentional and are certainly not strategic. The Ministry of Health has assumed that a constant share of health spending will be devoted to the wage bill in the coming years. Given that health spending is projected to increase and the overall wage bill is not, this assumption implies that the share of the overall public sector wage bill going to health will need to continue to increase. It is important that the ministry be prepared to make a good case as to why these additional resources are needed.

Major inefficiencies exist in the institutional arrangements for recruiting health workers into the public sector. But there are also very clear, demonstrated quick wins to address the problems. Despite the acknowledged staffing shortage, there are lengthy delays—up to 10 months—in filling vacant posts. One factor is the capacity of the PSC. A total of about 40 staff are responsible for recruiting the entire civil service—around 190,000 employees. This lack of capacity within the PSC presents an obvious bottleneck in the recruitment process. Time targets are included in the performance contracts of some of the key actors involved, and these targets should be monitored and enforced.

Currently, staff members are recruited to the Ministry of Health and then posted to a particular facility. There is no regular monitoring of whether staff members remain at that facility once they are posted there. When health workers leave their post, the highly centralized and time-consuming process for filling vacancies leads to long delays. The EHP has solved this problem. Decentralized recruitment, tying of salary payments to specific facilities and not to specific health workers, and improved monitoring of staff members have led to dramatic improvements in staffing levels in areas where the program was implemented.

Allowances make up a significant portion of total wages but do not provide incentives for good performance. In particular, the housing allowance, which comprises at least 20 percent of the total wage bill, plays a major role in driving pay differentials across regions in the opposite direction of what is needed to attract staff in remote areas. The hardship allowance is not large enough to compensate for this differential.

Promotion policy is not fully adhered to. The process is perceived as being opaque and slow, resulting in backlogs and low staff morale.

The Emergency Hiring Program has demonstrated that success is possible. The MOH can dramatically reduce the time it takes to fill posts and to reduce the opportunities for corruption in the process. Simple things such as computerizing the process and improving access to information have had dramatic results. Current recruitment policies, as well as the current incentive structure for health workers (salary, allowance schemes, and promotion and transfer policies), are not conducive to addressing geographic distribution and staff performance. But clear solutions have been demonstrated to address these issues also.

Notes

1. An exception exists for casual labor funded from others sources, such as income generated from fees.
2. Both Treasury Circular 28/2004 and the guidelines for preparing sector budgets in the 2005 and 2006 Budget Outlook Paper instruct line ministries to base the wage bill budget on current authorized establishment and any new recruitment will be allowed only following Treasury confirmation of availability of funding (Kenya Ministry of Finance 2006).
3. The Constituency Development Fund finances the creation of 1,000 (600 in 2007/08) new health facilities. These facilities will require about 3,000 extra health workers. The Ministry of Health is responsible for staffing these facilities.
4. Because of effective advocacy, mainly by provincial medical officers, most of these interns were in fact given jobs, even though the jobs had not been budgeted for.
5. Part of the PSC's mission is to provide a steady supply of staff members to government institutions.
6. In some cases, the allowance is used to service a mortgage that would not be affordable on a person's basic salary.
7. In general, it is much more difficult to carry out private practice in remote rural areas than in urban areas because of the sparseness of the population and the much lower level of disposable income.
8. It is not known how well regulated the policy restricting private practice by government employees in urban areas is, so this factor may also reduce the ability of the policy to act as an incentive.

References

Ambrose, Soren. 2006. "Preserving Disorder: IMF Policies and Kenya's Health Care Crisis." Global Policy Forum, New York. http://www.globalpolicy.org/socecon/bwi-wto/imf/2006/0601imfhealth.htm.

Andrews, David. 2007. "IMF Supportive of Health and Education in Kenya." Letter to the *Daily Nation*, Nairobi, December 13. http://www.imf.org/external/np/vc/2007/121307.htm.

Bor, Mark K. Arap. 2006. "Managing the Public Sector Wage Bill within a Harmonized Remuneration System: The Case of Kenya's Public Service." Paper presented at the Commonwealth Advanced Seminar Wellington, Nairobi, February 20–March 3.

Fedelino, Annalisa, Gerd Schwartz, and Marijn Verhoeven. 2006. "Aid Scaling Up: Do Wage Bill Ceilings Stand in the Way?" IMF Working Paper 06/106, International Monetary Fund, Washington, DC. http://www.imf.org/external/pubs/ft/wp/2006/wp06106.pdf.

IMF (International Monetary Fund). 2003. "Kenya: 2003 Article IV Consultation—Staff Report; Staff Supplement; Public Information Notice on the Executive Board Discussion; and Statement by the Executive Director for Kenya." IMF Country Report 03/199, IMF, Washington, DC. http://www.imf.org/external/pubs/ft/scr/2003/cr03199.pdf.

Kenya Ministry of Finance. 2006. "Budget Outlook Paper, 2006/7–2008/9." Kenya Ministry of Finance, Nairobi.

———. 2007a. "Budget Outlook Paper, 2007/08–2009/10." Kenya Ministry of Finance, Nairobi.

———. 2007b. "The Medium Term Budget Strategy Paper, 2007/08–2009/10." Kenya Ministry of Finance, Nairobi.

Kenya Ministry of Health. 2005a. "Human Resource Mapping and Verification Exercise." Kenya Ministry of Health, Nairobi.

———. 2005b. "The Second Kenya National Health Sector Strategic Plan (NHSSP II), 2005–2010." Kenya Ministry of Health, Nairobi. http://www.health.go.ke/hpdcon.htm.

———. 2006a. "Human Resources for Health Strategic Plan, 2006/7–2009/10." Kenya Ministry of Health, Nairobi.

———. 2006b. "Norms and Standards for Health Service Delivery." Kenya Ministry of Health, Nairobi.

———. 2007a. "Health Sector Working Group Report (MTEF 2007/8–2009/10)." Kenya Ministry of Health, Nairobi. http://www.treasury.go.ke/downloads/HEALTH_SECTOR_REPORT_2007%20_DRAFT_.pdf.

———. 2007b. "Public Expenditure Review, 2007." Kenya Ministry of Health, Nairobi.

Odundo, Paul, and John W. Wachira. 2004. "District Human Resource Needs Assessment: Draft Report of the Improved District Personnel Management Team." Health Sector Reform Secretariat, Kenya Ministry of Health, Nairobi.

WEMOS Foundation. 2005. "Budget Ceiling and Health: The Kenya Case Study." WEMOS Foundation, Amsterdam.

World Bank. 2007. *World Development Indicators 2007.* Washington, DC: World Bank.

CHAPTER 3

Background Country Study for Zambia

Health is a major priority for the government of Zambia. Not only is this priority outlined in the latest national policy document—the Fifth National Development Plan (NDP)—but it is also reflected in the government's future spending plans. As outlined in the latest Medium-Term Expenditure Framework (MTEF), social sector spending on health, education, and water and sanitation is one of the government's primary public spending priorities (Zambia Ministry of Finance and National Planning 2007). This policy represents a shift from the trend that saw total expenditure on health decline from US$24 million in 1997 to US$18 million in 2005, as well as a reduction in total health expenditure as a percentage of gross domestic product (GDP) from 6 percent in 1997 to 1.5 percent in 2005 (Fifth NDP).

Within the health sector, human resources for health (HRH) issues are a key priority. The National Health Strategic Plan (Zambia Ministry of Health 2005) recognizes that the availability of skilled human resources in adequate numbers is critical for realizing the sector's mission to deliver quality and accessible health services. The worsening human resource situation, which has kept the available workforce at 50 percent of the required levels, has also been identified as a pivotal constraint to the scaling up of health services. In 2004, the government of Zambia set up a task force to examine the situation, highlight key constraints, and make recommendations on strategies to address this issue. These recommendations have been incorporated in the Human Resources for Health Strategic Plan.

The Health Wage Bill in Zambia

It is important to understand the history of recent reforms before turning to the analysis. In 1995, following the decentralization reforms Zambia established the Central Board of Health (CBOH), hospital management boards, and district health boards. The impetus for these reforms was the belief that greater efficiency could be achieved by creating an internal market of various providers. As a result, the Ministry of Health (MOH) was split into two entities to separate provider and purchasing functions. The former function was delegated to the newly created CBOH, whereas the MOH was left with the residual functions of formulation of health policy, legislation, donor coordination, and monitoring of the health status and services. The CBOH carried out its function of providing health services by coordinating and regulating health boards at the district level, including their human resource management. The health boards (which were appointed by and served at the discretion of the minister of health) were responsible for managing hospitals and providing health services (Jeppsson and Okuonzi 2000).

The intention of these reforms was to delink all government health employees, except a skeleton MOH staff at headquarters, transferring all employment contracts to the health boards. However, because of poor coordination, fiscal constraints, and negotiating problems with unions, the government of Zambia backtracked on this reform process and abolished the health boards in 2006.

The failure of the delinking attempts and the reintegration of the health boards into the MOH led to even greater uncertainty for health workers and increased administrative burdens for the government officials who had to make sense of the new system. In Zambia, the difficulty in providing quality health services and increasing staffing levels has persisted. The health care system has been weakened by the inadequate number of personnel in vital areas of the health sector, including an insufficient total number of health workers in absolute terms, the inequitable distribution of health personnel, and the attrition of highly trained health workers, according to the Fifth NDP (2006–10).

Budget for the Public Sector Wage Bill

From 2000 to 2003, Zambia experienced a sharp increase in the public sector wage bill. The public sector wage bill remained relatively stable at 5 to 6 percent of GDP throughout the 1990s. This ratio was 5.9 percent in 2000, and by 2003 it had grown to 8.4 percent (figure 3.1). Furthermore, the government of Zambia calculated that 47 percent of domestic revenue was being used to remunerate civil servants (excluding housing allowances and salaries and wages paid by grant-aided institutions) (Zambia Ministry of Finance and National Planning 2003). This left few resources to finance service delivery and other poverty reduction programs, leading to an increased reliance on donor resources. Such a trend was deemed unsustainable.

To contain the increasing wage bill, the government of Zambia, in concert with the International Monetary Fund (IMF), made sustainable reductions in public sector wages as a percentage of GDP. Not only did the public sector wage bill increase dramatically, but it also well overran its budget in 2003, raising concerns of international donors and prohibiting Zambia from concluding its Poverty Reduction and Growth Facility (PRGF) program with the IMF (IMF 2004). The IMF instead put into place a Staff Monitored Program as an interim measure and consequently concluded a PRGF arrangement covering 2004 to 2006. In the previous PRGF arrangement, the IMF urged the government of Zambia to control the public sector wage bill; however, official conditionality on the wage bill was not included. Despite the wording in official documents, key

Figure 3.1   Public Sector Wage Bill as a Share of GDP, 1990–2008

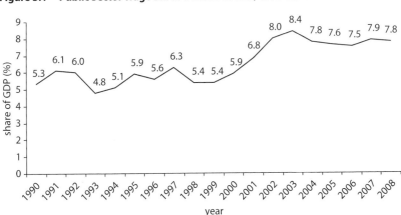

Sources: IMF 2007a, 2008; World Bank 2001.

informants have indicated that many in the government viewed this hiring freeze as a conditionality of IMF lending. The wage ceilings were set to accommodate the concrete hiring plans in the health and education sectors. However, compliance with this exemption of health and education was difficult to enforce or monitor during the implementation period because of a lack of adequate monitoring systems (Goldsbrough and Cheelo 2007).

After the problems of budget overruns in 2003, the government of Zambia made strides toward improving the fiscal discipline of the public sector wage bill and bringing it in line with budgetary realities and IMF guidelines. Targets were set to limit the amount spent on the wage bill as a percentage of GDP to 8.2 percent by 2004, 7.9 percent by 2005, and 7.6 percent by 2006 (Zambia Ministry of Finance and National Planning 2003). The government succeeded in bringing its public sector wage bill under control and in line with its set policy, as represented in figure 3.1, where the public sector wage bill decreased from 8.4 percent of GDP in 2003 to 7.8 percent of GDP in 2004. This decreasing trend continued until 2006, and the wage bill was projected to be 7.9 percent and 7.8 percent of GDP, respectively, for 2007 and 2008.

As of 2005, Zambia had a large public sector wage bill relative to other countries in the region. As a percentage of GDP, the public sector wage bill within Zambia was 7.6 percent (figure 3.2). This percentage is relatively high in comparison with that of other Sub-Saharan Africa countries. Figure 3.3 illustrates that Zambia's public sector wage bill was 29.8 percent of total government expenditure in 2005, which was about average in relation to other Sub-Saharan African countries.

The reductions in the public sector wage bill trend are in line with the quantitative performance criteria included in Zambia's PRGF arrangements with the IMF since 2003. Since then, wage bill ceilings have been targeted at approximately 8 percent of GDP (Goldsbrough and Cheelo 2007). These ceilings are indicative benchmarks and not formal performance criteria. Additionally, Zambia has to provide to the IMF on a monthly basis and by budget head the following data: (a) the number of all employees in the central government for each budget head; (b) the basic salary, the allowances, and any other personnel emoluments released during the month; (c) the arrears incurred during the month on the basic salary, the allowances, and any other personnel emoluments; and (d) the number of employees retrenched and the corresponding retrenchment costs (IMF 2007b). The purpose of this increased level of reporting is to ensure that Zambia continues to exercise fiscal prudence in the management of its

Figure 3.2 Public Sector Wage Bill as a Share of GDP, by Country, 2005

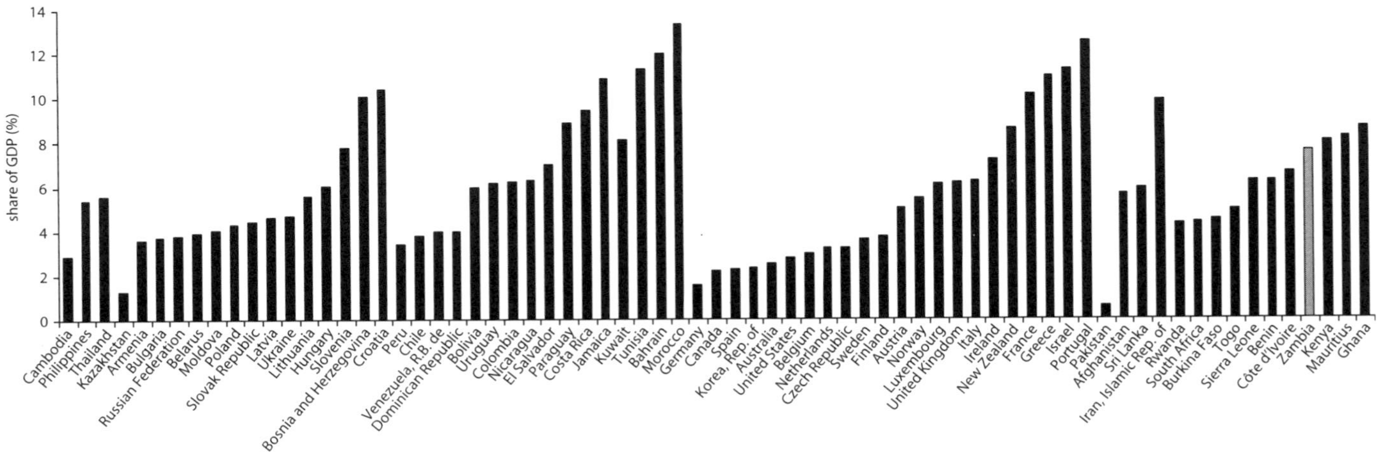

Source: World Bank 2007.

Figure 3.3   Public Sector Wage Bill as a Share of Government Expenditure, by Country, 2005

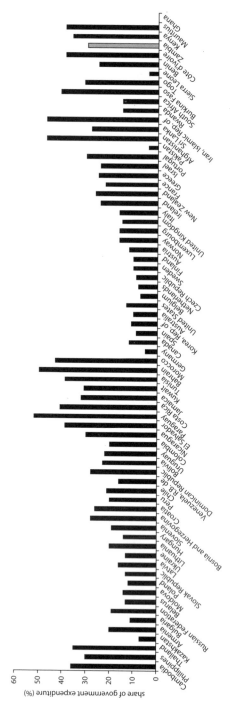

Source: World Bank 2007.

public sector wage bill and does not revert to its previous budget overruns. Interviews with key public sector officials reveal the general recognition that increased management of the public sector wage bill was necessary. Although the government of Zambia brought down the public sector wage bill as a share of GDP, it did not do so as a share of overall government expenditure. Figure 3.4 shows the steady increasing trend from 2000 to 2007, with the public sector wage bill as a share of government expenditure growing from 19 percent to 34.4 percent. The trend is projected to change in 2008, with the public sector wage bill as a share of government expenditure slightly dropping to 33.0 percent.

Beginning in 2000, the public sector wage bill expanded rapidly. At the recommendation of the IMF, a hiring freeze was introduced in 2002 to contain the wage bill, but doctors and nurses were specifically excluded.

In 2001, a review of the salary scale for all civil service employees was conducted; recommendations were issued in March 2002 and were approved by the cabinet in 2002. The main recommendations were to reduce the number of salary grades, decompress the salaries, and consolidate some allowances into salaries. In the negotiations, the unions agreed to the decompression but refused the consolidation of allowances into salaries, leading to higher allowances. (The allowances were fixed percentages of salaries, which hence increased with the new decompressed salaries.)

These higher allowances and salary increases were not budgeted for and resulted in overruns in the 2003 budget.[1] In response, another hiring freeze was put in place, and the IMF introduced measures to keep the wage bill within the agreed limit of 8 percent of GDP.

Figure 3.4   Public Sector Wage Bill as a Share of Government Expenditure, 1990–2008

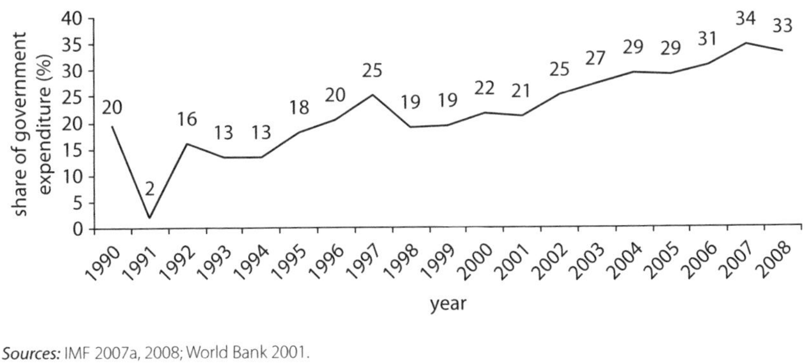

Sources: IMF 2007a, 2008; World Bank 2001.

The hiring freeze affected the entire public service except additional health workers and teachers. Health workers were hired through the newly created health boards. The Ministry of Education was allowed to hire to replace teachers who were dying, retiring, resigning, or migrating. To fill any other post, the responsible permanent secretary would apply to the Public Service Reform Program Steering Committee, chaired by the secretary to the cabinet, for permission to hire. In most cases, this permission was not granted for nontechnical and nonprofessional personnel.

Budget for the Health Sector Wage Bill

The process for determining the budget for the health sector wage bill begins with the overall NDP. The strategic focus of the Fifth NDP is economic infrastructure and human resource development. The NDP outlines the government's overall wage bill policy and sets priority areas, including reference to health and education as key investment areas (Zambia Ministry of Finance and National Planning 2005).

The MOH has developed an HRH strategy that contains alternative costed wage bill scenarios. In response to the exposure of the human resource crisis (Zambia Ministry of Health 2005), the president of the Republic of Zambia instructed the MOH to develop the Human Resources for Health Strategic Plan for 2006–10. Using World Health Organization (WHO) recommendations on staff-to-population ratios (for example, 1:5,000 and 1:700 for doctors and nurses, respectively), the plan suggested that the current staff establishment[2] would have to increase from 23,176 to 49,360. In fact, the establishment was finally approved by the MOH in September 2006 at about 51,000.[3] Although this increase has been approved, not all the posts have been funded by the Ministry of Finance and National Planning; however, the government plans to fund all posts, in phases, upon Treasury approval. For 2008, the number of funded positions was increased to 30,883. This figure gives plenty of room for expansion in the long term, but the HRH strategic plan provides a more realistic approach to expansion in the period up to 2010. It gives three costed scenarios, ranging from increases from a base figure of 23,162 to between 25,796 and 25,856 (that is, a maximum of 11.6 percent) by 2011 or a maximum average annual increase of 1.9 percent.

The process of determining the budget for the health wage bill of the MOH is in line with the general budget cycle for the operational budget, which is mainly determined by the Ministry of Finance and National Planning, as described in table 3.1. Line ministries are required to prepare budgets in accordance with specific guidelines issued annually by the Ministry of Finance and National Planning. These guidelines are closely

Table 3.1   Main Stages and Actors in the Budget Planning Cycle

Approximate timing	Step	Actors
April–May	• Guidelines for line ministries prepared	Ministry of Finance and Planning
June–July	• Planning cycle launched • Provincial teams sent to MOH Human Resource Department for briefing on priorities based on the Fifth NDP and the National Health Strategic Plan; broad ceilings from the MTEF provided	MOH headquarters and provinces
	• Action plan (not personnel emoluments budget) developed by provincial offices, working with districts and hospitals	Provinces, districts, and other units
September–October	• Budget ceilings provided to line ministries	Ministry of Finance and Planning
October–November	• Negotiations (including on personnel emoluments) held and revisions made	MOH headquarters, provinces, and districts
November–December	• Budget meetings held with line ministries	Ministry of Finance and Planning
December	• Budget set • Budget printed in Yellow Book • Provisional warrant to spend issued by president	Ministry of Finance and Planning
January	• Financial year started	
January–March	• Ministerial brief prepared for submission for parliamentary approval (which takes over from presidential warrant)	Line ministries
March	• Budget approved	Parliament
When required	• Supplementary budget developed and submitted	MOH

Sources: Interviews during the study.

linked and reflect the expenditure priorities outlined in the government's MTEF, which is issued annually along with the coming year's budget. The MTEF outlines revenue projections and provides three-year expenditure envelopes for each line ministry as well as the public sector wage bill budget. These projections are made on the basis of the budget envelope and reflect the government's strategy concerning the public sector wage bill. The MTEF specifically describes the number of additional employees that can be hired in each sector. For example, the 2007–09 MTEF states that 5,715 medical personnel and 15,000 teachers will be recruited over the medium term. To reflect this increase in teachers and medical personnel, the MTEF makes allocations of K 89.0 billion, K 120.0 billion, and K 132.0 billion in 2007, 2008, and 2009, respectively.

In practice, actual budgetary allocations differ from those outlined in the MTEF. Specifically, although the public sector wage bill ceiling is adhered to, the allocations of additional wage bill resources across different ministries often differ from those outlined in the MTEF. The size of the public sector wage bill appears to be much more of a priority to the Ministry of Finance and National Planning than how it is divided across sectors. Thus, the budgeting process becomes more of a year-by-year negotiation, determined by the cost of current staffing levels and whatever increment in staffing numbers can be negotiated, than a coherent, predictable three-year process. For example, the 2007–09 MTEF stated that additional health workers (about 5,715) were to be hired over the medium term, but in fact the initial budgetary allocation from the Ministry of Finance and National Planning for the health wage bill in 2007 was less than that in 2006. This situation led to negotiations between the Ministry of Health and the Ministry of Finance and National Planning where the health sector successfully negotiated an increase in the allocation. In 2007, the MOH was able to negotiate an additional 1,905 new recruits, or in financial terms, an increase from K 294 billion for 2006 to K 382 million for 2007. Recently, the MOH was granted authorization by the Treasury and the Ministry of Finance and National Planning to hire more staff to bring the projected total number of public sector health workers to about 30,883 in 2008 from 26,523 in 2007 (Zambia Ministry of Health 2008).

Actual salaries paid to staff are not always captured under the personnel emoluments line item of the budget. Therefore, the budgetary guideline that personnel emoluments should not exceed 8 percent of GDP does not take into account all wage-related remuneration. In the health sector, certain institutions (grant-aided institutions) receive block grants from the MOH, from which salaries and allowances are paid. These block grants are not recorded as personnel emoluments and therefore are not captured. Second, before the reintegration of the health boards into the ministry, some of the boards were paying salaries and top-ups from their operational grant, which again were not captured as personnel emoluments. For example, CBOH's approximately 300 employees were recorded in nonwage expenditure because they were paid from grants.

The magnitude of the effect these off–wage bill expenditures have on the public sector wage bill is unclear. According to key stakeholder interviews with the Ministry of Finance and National Planning and Ministry of Health, these expenditures do not significantly affect the public sector wage bill. However, the ability to pay salaries and top-ups out of the grants allows these institutions to circumvent the implicit wage bill ceilings. The additional expenditure grant-aided institutions were able to allocate to personnel emoluments often came at the expense of operations and service delivery in the health sector. The discovery that a far greater proportion of the grants was going toward paying personnel emoluments than intended was considered a contributing factor to the unsustainability of the health board system.[4]

Clearly, overall weaknesses in public sector management processes need to be addressed. The MTEF is supposed to be the tool to guide sector budget allocations; however, in practice, it is only indicative. The Ministry of Finance and National Planning decides on the MOH's resources allocation on the basis of revenue availability each year. Not only does this situation create some degree of uncertainty, but the final allocation also depends on the ability of the MOH to make its case to the Ministry of Finance and National Planning. Because inefficiencies in the health sector in the past year prevented the MOH from filling all the funded vacancies on time—that is, within the budget year—this method of resource allocation is increasingly difficult to sustain.

In addition, the timing of the budget allocation process is an issue. The budgeting process takes about a year, and the budget is not approved until March—three months into the fiscal year (which begins on January 1). In effect, three months of complete uncertainty on the wage bill budget make hiring and other human resource management difficult.

Results of the Wage Bill Budgeting Process

The health sector accounted for an increasing share of the overall wage bill until 2000. Following the fiscal controls in 2001, this trend was reversed, but this decrease does not necessarily indicate nonprioritization of the health sector. Available data show that in the past decade, health was prioritized in the public sector wage bill. From approximately 1994 until 2000, the proportion of the public sector wage bill that went to health increased continuously until it spiked at 14 percent in 2000 (see figure 3.5). According to key stakeholders interviewed, factors that contributed to this spike include the integration that occurred within this period of health workers from various health boards and other agencies, such as mines and

Figure 3.5   Health Bill as a Share of Public Sector Wage Bill, 1990–2007

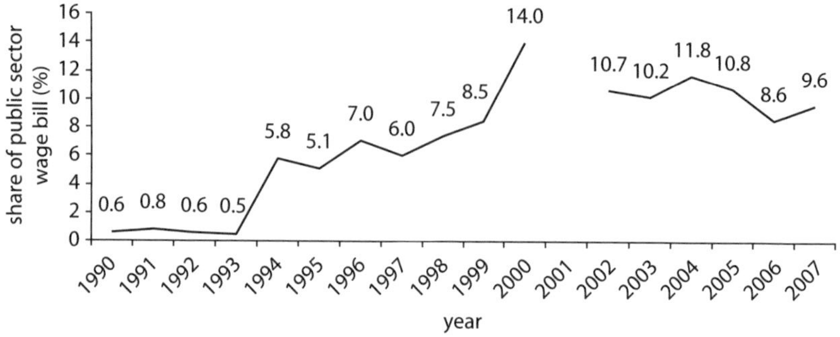

Sources: World Bank 2001, 2008.

Note: Data are unavailable for 2001. Health expenditure includes government of Zambia funding and the basket of funds various donors provide; however, it does not include overall donor funding. When donor funding is included, the proportion of health expenditure dedicated to wages falls, because most of the donor funding is used to fund service delivery and nonwage expenditures. For instance, in 2006, if just government of Zambia funding is considered, 57 percent of health expenditure is dedicated to personnel emoluments, but if all donor funding, including vertical funds and the basket, is taken into account, this ratio falls to 22 percent. The government of Zambia has discretion over donors' basket funding, and therefore it is included in this graph.

faith-based organizations, into the health wage bill. During this period, the increasing recruitment in the preceding years had not been effectively monitored and integrated into the official list of government health workers.

The health wage bill was brought down and has since remained at about 10 percent of the public sector wage bill. Several factors contributed to this apparent decline in the health wage bill relative to the public sector wage bill. The first factor has to do with accounting mechanisms. Several grant-aided institutions that were initially put on the payroll were subsequently delinked and reverted to their previous status. Under that status, salaries and other personnel emoluments were paid out of the block grants, which did not appear in the budget as personnel emoluments. The Ministry of Finance and National Planning could not accurately determine what proportion of such grants went to wages.[5] Second, in 2006, the boards of health were dissolved, and the staff of these boards was brought back into the civil service and subjected to its terms of service, which are less generous. Some reduction in the health wage bill, therefore, was expected.

Grant-aided institutions were able to hire non–civil service employees and, in turn, were able to avoid wage bill restrictions. Grant-aided agencies (including the CBOH before its abolition) used block grants to finance wages, enabling the health sector to circumvent any restrictions or limits on hiring caused by public sector wage bill ceilings. These grants were also used by the health boards to top-up civil servant salaries so they were more comparable with the generous salaries paid to employees hired directly by the health boards. Figure 3.6 illustrates government health expenditure as a share of total government expenditure and the health wage bill as a share of health expenditure.

After a period of remaining relatively flat, the wage bill as a percentage of health expenditure increased significantly in 2001 before stabilizing and leveling off in 2004 and declining in 2005. Some of the reasons for the initial increase include newly negotiated wages, salary decompression, and integration of employees of grant-aided institutions into the civil service. Second, the denominator (government health expenditure) was not increasing significantly because of the smaller increase in nonwage expenditure, especially given that external resources for health, primarily donor funding, increased significantly and were used in large part to finance nonwage expenditure.

As illustrated in figure 3.6, health expenditure as a share of government expenditure, after a steady upward trend in the 1990s, has been declining since 2000. It appears to be leveling off at 10 percent and is projected to increase. Zambia is committed to raising government expenditure on health to 15 percent of the total, the target set at the special 2001 summit in Abuja, Nigeria, which was devoted specifically to addressing the challenges of HIV/AIDS, tuberculosis, and other related infectious diseases.

Figure 3.6   Health Expenditure as a Share of Government Expenditure and Health Wage Bill as a Share of Health Expenditure, 1990–2009

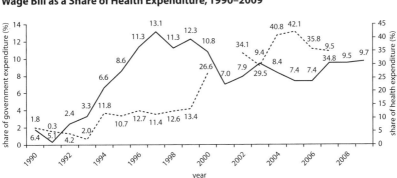

Sources: IMF 2007a, 2008; World Bank 2001, 2008.

While the size of government health expenditure relative to total expenditure was decreasing, money from external sources was increasing. Figure 3.7 shows that, whereas general government expenditure on health as a percentage of total health expenditure went from 54.7 percent to 50.3 percent during 2001 to 2005, external resources on health as a percentage of total health expenditure increased from 14.1 percent to 53.4 percent within the same time frame. Some of the external sources of funding were channeled through the government, however, and thus captured in the government health expenditure numbers.

The process for determining the budget for nonwage health expenditure is divorced from the process for determining the wage bill. The health expenditure reductions during 2001 to 2004 were mainly attributable to nonsalary expenditures. Beginning in 2006, this trend is projected to change as health spending increases. The share of health spending devoted to the wage bill increased from 34 percent to 42 percent. This increase suggests either a deliberate decision within the health sector to minimize staffing reductions or indicates lack of MOH flexibility in reducing staffing levels because of the desire to meet the Abuja targets.

Despite the wage bill constraints, the health sector continued hiring, both directly into the payroll and through contracts paid out of block grants. Figure 3.8 illustrates the hiring levels by the Ministry of Health from 1999 to 2007.

Figure 3.7   Expenditure on Health, 1996–2005

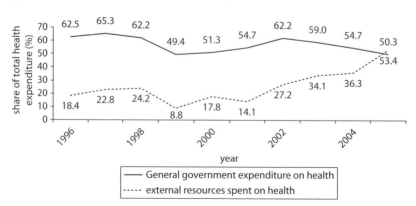

Source: WHO Zambia National Health Accounts.

Figure 3.8   Number of Ministry of Health Staff Appointed, 1999–2007

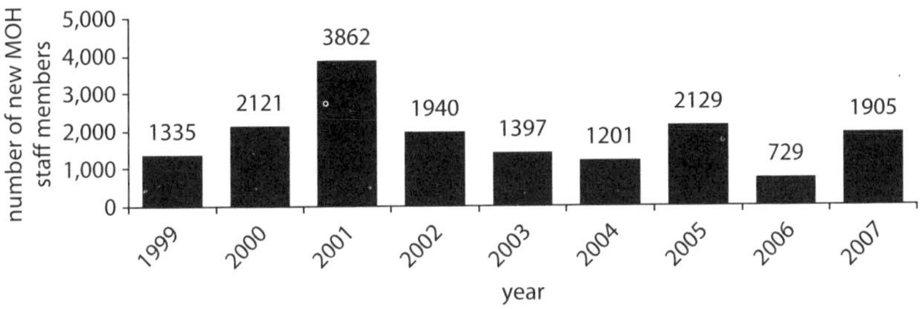

Source: Zambia MOH payroll 2006.

Table 3.2   MOH Medium-Term Expenditure Framework 2004–10

	Amount (K billion)						
Type of expenditure	2004 budget	2005 budget	2006 ceiling	2007 budget	2008 ceiling	2009 projections	2010 projections
Personnel emoluments and other emolument-related expenditure ceilings	234	271	294	392	442	511	577
Of which net recruitment	0	32	14	30	24	24	24

Source: Zambia Ministry of Finance and National Planning 2003, 2004, 2005, 2006, 2007.

Table 3.2 shows that, consistent with the HRH strategy and the government's prioritization of health, hiring is projected to remain at a relatively constant rate through 2010.

The Ministry of Health's capacity to implement its wage bill budget is limited, despite the critical shortage of health workers, demonstrating that the resource envelope is not the only constraint to scaling up the health workforce in Zambia. The capacity of the ministry to execute its wage bill budget appears low. In 2006, the MOH spent 50.13 percent of its allocated wage bill, and in 2007, it executed only 69.81 percent of its total wage bill budget. In contrast, the Ministry of Education implemented 94.23 percent and 102.03 percent of its wage bill budget in 2006 and 2007, respectively. This finding points either to an intrinsic inefficiency in the health system, leading to the inability to recruit for funded positions, or to widespread limitations in capacity at the MOH.

Public Sector Employment of Health Workers

Background to the Current Employment Situation

The way health workers have been employed over the past 10 years has changed several times. In 1992, a restructuring of the health sector began as part of a decentralization program in which key management responsibilities and resources were devolved to the district level. As part of this restructuring, parallel but complementary organizational structures were introduced: (a) popular structures to encourage broader participation in decision making and (b) technical structures to strengthen management capacity at such decentralized levels. At the national level, these popular structures included the CBOH; at the district and province levels, the district health boards and hospital management boards; and at the community level and health center level, the Neighborhood Health Committees and Health Centre Committees. These technical structures included the CBOH management teams at the national level, the District Health Management Teams (DHMTs) at district level, the Hospital Management Teams at level 2 and 3 hospitals, and the Provincial Health Offices under the CBOH.

As a result of the restructuring, Medical Services Act No. 14 of 1985 (the law that previously governed health workers in Zambia) was repealed and replaced by National Health Services Act No. 22 of 1995. A key component of these reforms of 1992 and the new National Health Services Act of 1995 was the proposed delinking of service provision from the MOH and transfer of such functions (along with respective staff) to the health boards. The CBOH was established under section 11 of this new Health Services Act to take over the service provision functions in the health sector. The district and hospital health boards were established to grant more autonomy to provider institutions. The MOH was to be reformed into a lean body that retained its roles in policy making, legislation, donor coordination, budgeting, resource mobilization, advocacy, and oversight of the CBOH. As a result, the ministry was downsized from 220 employees to about 90. The CBOH was staffed with approximately 300 managers, administrative staff members, and health officers, all of whom were employed directly by CBOH and were not part of the overall civil service.

The conditions of service for workers in these boards were different (and often more favorable) than those of the civil service. The initial plan was that eventually all health staff members (except a few who would be retained in the MOH) would be delinked from the civil service and employed directly by the health boards. This structure would allow facilities to fully manage their own staff in line with the decentralization of other management functions and would also allow the CBOH to provide salaries and conditions more in line with what was available in the local labor market without being constrained by the wider public service statutes.

However, the proposed delinkage never took place completely for the following reasons. First, the delinking was supposed to have been preceded by the retirement of the civil servants from the MOH before they joined the staff of the boards of health. This early retirement would have had significant financial implications under the rules for permanent and pensionable staff, which the Ministry of Health could not afford. Second, the terms of the delinkage were unclear, creating significant anxiety among the unions—especially the Civil Service Union of Zambia—because the terms of service under the boards were not yet formally instituted. The applications by the boards to the Cabinet Office were never approved. Third, the Ministry of Health feared losing health workers if they did not find the terms of the delinkage favorable—a major cause of concern in a country with significant human resources for health shortages. A compromise was reached in which the ministry's staff was considered to be on "secondment" or "attachment" to the boards.

This outcome implied a dual responsibility status, where the workers were still civil servants under the MOH and government statutes but were being directly managed by the health boards. In certain boards, such as the CBOH, the terms of service were better, and to compensate, the seconded staff was paid salary top-ups by the CBOH.[6] In addition to the seconded staff, the health boards could also hire staff members on a contractual basis on their own terms.

The funds that were allocated to the boards came in two forms: (a) block grants, which were not earmarked, and (b) a basket of funds from a pool that was earmarked by particular programs (for example, programs for HIV/AIDS). The block grants were also used to hire staff members on temporary contracts. Such staff members would not show up on the personnel emoluments for the MOH, nor would the top-ups paid to the secondees, because these funds were from grants.

The CBOH carried out its provision function by coordinating and regulating health boards at the district and hospital levels, including their human resource management. The hospital management boards were responsible for managing hospitals and providing health services. These health boards were appointed by and served at the discretion of the minister of health (Jeppsson and Okuonzi 2000). As part of this structure, the DHMTs prepared annual plans and budgets, which were derived from inputs from communities and health centers. This information was aggregated, approved by the district health boards, and then submitted to the CBOH for approval.

Between 2002 and 2004, the government cut back on staff across the civil service using first voluntary then compulsory redundancy strategies. It also constrained and at times even froze all recruitment, including the replacement of staff members who left or retired. Having gained some autonomy over their budgets as a result of the health reforms, many hospitals and districts compensated for this freeze on official recruitment by employing both professional and support staff members directly, using a combination of some of the operational budget and income from user fees to fund the posts.[7]

In March 2001, following the restructuring of the Ministry of Health and in accordance with the issuance of Treasury Authority 1 of 2001 (February 26, 2001), all health worker positions in the ministry were abolished; hence, the MOH did not have any positions or terms of service for health workers. Interestingly, in March 2001, the salary scales of all health workers were supposed to be changed to the health board scales (which, though higher than the civil service scales, had not yet been officially approved). Such was the confusion surrounding the delinkage process.

Therefore, there were now three categories of health workers in the public sector: (a) the civil servants (some who were in the civil service and others who were seconded to the respective health boards and various faith-based organizations), (b) workers employed directly by the health boards, and (c) health workers in grant-aided institutions.[8] The civil servants seconded to the boards of health were still being paid for the most part by the MOH according to civil service statutes.

In 2006, the Ministry of Health decided to relink the ministry and the CBOH for the following reasons. First was the realization that the anticipated delinking of all health workers was going to be very expensive and unsustainable, given budgetary constraints. Second was a perception that service delivery did not improve significantly. Moreover, the ministry felt it had very little control over the situation, given the level of autonomy granted to the CBOH under the reforms. Third was duplication of functions between the ministry and CBOH, whose respective new roles were not fully implemented. Fourth, the confusion created by the dual reporting structures of the civil servants, who were now employed under old civil service norms that no longer existed and managed by the boards of health with service norms that had not been approved (except for the terms of the contracts they had with their contractual staff), made this system an administrative nightmare for the MOH.

With the gradual reversal of the delinkage, culminating in the abolition of the CBOH in 2006, the Ministry of Health created a new establishment with terms of service and began moving all its employees back onto the government payroll. This changeover has been achieved for nearly all technical staff members, but some support staff members have still to be transferred. The exception is a small number of health workers who are employed by local government municipalities and the University Teaching Hospital.

As civil servants, health workers are part of a standard pay structure with common conditions of service with minor variations in terms of allowances and conditions of service. The following sections describe how health workers are currently recruited, deployed, and managed in the public sector.

Creating Funded Posts in the Health Sector

The number and type of posts that can be filled by the MOH is determined by the establishment. Until the past few years, recruitment into positions by facilities was somewhat ad hoc and not based on any establishment. In 2006, an establishment of 51,414 positions were created that take into account various factors, such as core functions at each level of service delivery, projections of population growth, the basic health care package at each service delivery level, and the government's desire to improve health outcomes. To determine this establishment, the ministry, together with the Management Development Division, consults with the districts and the DHMTs to assess actual need in all facilities, taking into account the WHO recommendations. The cabinet then approves recommendations and forwards them to the Public Service Management Division (PSMD).

The creation of newly funded positions in the health sector does not rest entirely with the Ministry of Health. Creation of funded posts is based on a budget envelope determined by the Ministry of Finance and National Planning in consultation with the PSMD, the Management Development Division, and the MOH. Newly vacated positions also require the same approval process, which is in large part outside the purview of the MOH. The Ministry of Health is responsible for developing staffing requirements for the health sector. The PSMD is responsible for maintaining a list of approved (but not necessarily funded) posts (the establishment) for each line ministry that the cabinet has approved. Most health workers in the public sector in Zambia are part of a national civil service, so there is a single national establishment. Other public sector health workers are employed by other entities such as the security forces, which are not part of the establishment and are funded directly from the budget of that ministry.

Each year during the budgeting process, the government allocates additional resources for the public sector wage bill to different ministries. In the health sector, the additional resources are allocated as a lump sum in response to the request by the MOH, which is based on estimated additional human resource needs. These additional resources received by the Ministry of Health are used to fund new posts in the establishment as well as to finance promotions and salary increases. The MOH decides how this allocation will be made. Within this budget, the MOH also decides the skill mix and cadres of health workers to be recruited.

The process for filling recently vacated posts is cumbersome and involves coordination across many levels of government and agencies. It is thus prone to significant delays. A post that is already approved and funded may become vacant because an incumbent resigns or retires (early or at the statutory age), is transferred or dismissed, or suffers long-term sickness or death. If a person is seconded elsewhere or absconds, the post does not count as being vacant and therefore cannot be filled. This situation may cause a post to be blocked for a long time. Confirming that an existing post has become vacant involves a complicated process that is outlined in box 3.1.

As can be seen from box 3.1, the process of verifying a vacancy is both complex and time consuming even if things run smoothly. Because of poor controls in the past, information about a post becoming vacant has not always been communicated to managers who can take action to fill the posts. Sometimes, this situation allows the individual or others to continue to draw the salary as what is called a "ghost worker."[9]

Recruiting Health Workers in the Public Sector

The Ministry of Health has been unable to fill all funded positions within the establishment because of inefficiencies in the current system of recruitment of health workers.

Box 3.1

Confirming That an Existing Post Has Become Vacant

A detailed process is required in Zambia to confirm that an existing post has become vacant:

- First, the outgoing incumbent's details have to be removed from the payroll by a clerk in the district office on the Payroll Management and Establishment Control (PMEC) system. The PMEC system is currently centralized and located in the Public Service Management Department; therefore, the district clerk has to travel monthly to Lusaka to update the information. Delays may occur if such vacancies are not reported in a timely manner.

- A request to fill the vacancy is made by the facility in charge to the district office, which passes on the details to the provincial office, which, in turn, passes them on to the Directorate of Human Resources and Administration (DHR&A) at the MOH. Avoiding delays would require some proactivity on the part of the district and provincial human resource clerks.

- At the DHR&A, the requests are first reviewed by the director and then passed on to the chief human resource management officer. A manual process is used to (a) verify the existence of the post against the establishment and (b) verify that the post is funded in the current budget. An individual letter is then prepared and typed for the permanent secretary of health to send to the permanent secretary of the PSMD, requesting permission to fill the vacancy. The DHR&A, which only has three human resource officers, may handle up to 900 of these requests a year; thus, processing delays are not uncommon.

- The PSMD checks that the vacancy has been cleared on the PMEC system. This process applies to all ministries; hence delays might occur from a huge workload. Once the vacancy has been cleared, the permanent secretary of the PSMD writes to the permanent secretary of health with the approval to fill the vacancy.

Source: Interviews conducted during the study.

Recruitment of health workers into funded posts is managed centrally, with significant involvement of agencies outside the Ministry of Health. Before the reintegration of the health boards into the ministry, health facilities were allowed to hire health workers on a provisional basis as needed, with the expectation that they would be absorbed into the civil service. This process has since changed. Currently, recruitment can occur only into already funded positions.

Job advertisements typically do not specify the geographic location or type of facility where the vacancy is located. When the MOH receives Treasury authority to recruit positions for the coming year, it advertises against the cadres to create a pool of health workers to fill the funded positions. These advertised positions are not matched to specific vacancies. Deployment to specific positions occurs after recruitment. Therefore, candidates apply not knowing where they would be deployed and thus must be willing to accept deployment to any location in the country. Experience has shown that people posted to remote areas sometimes lasted only six months there. Recruitment consists mainly of checking relevant qualifications. Successful candidates are provided with a provisional letter of appointment,[10] requesting the individual to report to his or her place of work. Upon reporting for work, the individual then sends relevant papers and qualifications to the PSMD,[11] which then forwards these documents to the Public Service Commission (PSC) for approval.[12] This approval is a confirmation that the individual will become permanent and pensionable. For administrative staff members, the PSC is involved in the recruitment and selection process, which is far more complicated.[13]

Long delays occur in the current process of recruiting health workers into funded posts in the health sector (table 3.3), although the source of bureaucratic delays in this rather complex recruitment process is difficult to clearly identify; it seems multifaceted. One issue is the centralized hiring process, under which even filling recently vacated posts requires central approval from the PSMD, often resulting in delays in filling positions, given the numerous steps required and multiple levels of government involved in the process. In addition, the fact that health workers are no longer recruited on a rolling basis that is managed by the facility has made it less efficient. Recruitment into new positions now occurs only with the timing of budgetary allocations, which are not entirely predictable and are time bound by the fiscal year. For instance, in 2007, of the approximately 1,700 funded positions, the MOH was able to fill only 1,400 positions within the budgetary time frame, despite the obvious needs. Funding for 300 positions had to be returned to the Ministry of Finance and Planning.[14]

The distribution of health workers in Zambia displays imbalances. Disparities exist by region as well as between rural and urban areas. For

Table 3.3 MOH Staff Levels against Approved Establishment, 2004 and 2008

Cadre	2004 Approved establishment	2004 Staff in post	2004 Variance	2008 Approved establishment	2008 Staff in post	2008 Variance
Doctors	2,300	646	1,654	1,778	1,290	488
Nurses	16,732	6,096	10,636	14,053	8,165	5,888
Midwives	5,600	2,273	3,327	4,751	2,775	1,976
Clinical officers	4,000	1,161	2,839	3,737	2,657	1,080
Medical licentiates	n.s.	n.s.	n.s.	547	79	468
Pharmacy staff	162	108	54	1,238	693	545
Laboratory staff	1,560	417	1,143	1,403	697	706
Environmental health workers	1,640	803	837	2,555	1,276	1,279
Teaching staff	n.s.	n.s.	n.s.	422	237	185
Dental staff	633	56	577	n.s.	n.s.	n.s.
Physiotherapist staff	300	86	214	n.s.	n.s.	n.s.
Radiography staff	233	142	91	732	327	405
Other paramedical staff	6,000	320	5,680	1,379	485	894
Nutritionist	200	65	135	n.s.	n.s.	n.s.
Administrative staff	n.s.	n.s.	n.s.	7,769	3,952	3,817
Support staff	10,000	11,003	−1,003	11,040	8,250	2,790
Total	49,360	23,176	26,184	51,040	30,883	20,157

Source: Director of human resources, Zambia Ministry of Health, April 2008.
Note: n.s. = not specified in the establishment for the given year.

instance, in Lusaka, the doctor-to-population ratio is 1:6,247, compared with 1:65,763 in the Northern Province. Not surprisingly, poorer provinces have more severe HRH shortages.

Terms of Work in the Public Sector

Terms of work include tenure, remuneration, promotion, and termination and sanctioning.

Tenure. A shift toward consolidation of various types of health worker contracts has occurred, through which staff members have been incorporated into the civil service where applicable. Civil servants now constitute the majority of the categories of health workers in the MOH. Health workers in Zambia are divided into four categories, based on tenure:

- Permanent, pensionable staff members who are part of the overall civil service
- Contract staff members—that is, those still serving the remainder of their contracts as part of the recruitment under the health boards and permanent, pensionable staff members with three-year contracts under the Zambia health worker retention scheme, which applies to doctors (and is now extended to other health workers) willing to work in rural areas[15]
- Casual employees, who are usually administrative and ancillary workers
- Expatriate workers, who are paid for and employed by their sponsors from abroad

The number of expatriate health workers has been increasing.[16]

Part-time work is not normal in the civil service. However, it is used in the University Training Hospital, a semiautonomous institution, partly as a retention measure. It allows staff members to have secure jobs but also to work in the private sector to supplement government wages. Doctors are allowed to carry out private practice, but this work is expected to take place outside their civil service working hours. Apparently, this requirement is not tightly managed.

Since the abolition of the CBOH, most staff members working for the MOH are now civil servants and are therefore on permanent and pensionable contracts. Under the CBOH, many staff members in the headquarters and senior staff members at the province and district levels, as well as in larger hospitals, were on fixed-term contracts paid for from the government grant. With the abolition of the CBOH and health boards, most of these staff members were reabsorbed into the civil service. Some were allowed to run out the terms of their contracts before being offered the option of absorption into the civil service under civil service conditions. Preference was given to the professional staff. The use of short-term contracts is very limited and now applies mostly to retirees who are hired back into the service.

Under the health boards, facilities could employ staff on short-term contracts funded out of operational budgets and income from user fees. For example, Lusaka DHMT had funded 648 positions (188 professional and 460 support) by this means to supplement the approximately 2,100 staff members funded by the Treasury. Professional staff members on these short-term contracts usually expect to be hired as permanent and pensionable civil servants as posts become available. Support staff members usually do not have this opportunity because posts do not exist for them in the new establishment, which has emphasized professional rather than support posts.

This shift toward the use of permanent contracts has likely reduced an important incentive for overall staff performance. Managers have less control over the hiring process. They have also lost power over who is selected and the speed of the process. In addition, they find it more difficult to dismiss nonperforming workers and sometimes resort to simply taking on new staff members to do the work of the poor performers and absentees.

Remuneration. Health workers and medical doctors are paid on salary scales (Medical Salary Scale, or MSS, and Medical Doctor Salary Scale, or MDS, respectively) that are different from those of other civil servants (General Salary Scale, or GSS). Moreover, a significant part of the health staff's total remuneration is from allowances, which are not part of the personnel emoluments from the Ministry of Finance and Planning. Most staff members on the government payroll are placed according to job and grade on a single pay scale that is used across the public service. Remuneration of health workers is based on a civil service-wide pay scale and system of allowances; however, doctors and other health workers are paid on separate pay scales that exist only in the health sector. These pay scales are slightly higher than the equivalent GSS levels.

Therefore, three pay scales are relevant to workers in the health sector. They include the GSS pay scale, which applies to nonclinical managers and administrative personnel; the MSS, which applies to all medical workers, excluding medical doctors and pharmacists; and the MDS, which applies to doctors and pharmacists. Tables 3.4, 3.5, and 3.6 illustrate these pay scales in detail.

Allowances make up a significant proportion of the overall earnings of government workers. Various allowances apply to all civil servants, such as subsistence allowance, uniform upkeep, transport and baggage repatriation, settling, and rural and hardship allowances. Recruitment and retention allowances are paid to all graduate civil servants regardless

Table 3.4   General Salary Scale as of April 1, 2007

Scale	Minimum salary (K)	Maximum salary (K)	Example
GS01	73,438,728	80,362,152	Director
GS02	61,198,932	66,968,484	Deputy director
GS03	50,999,124	55,807,068	Assistant director
GS04	42,499,248	46,505,928	Principal subject specialist
GS05	35,416,056	38,754,936	Chief HRMO/HRDO
GS06	29,513,364	33,940,404	Senior subject specialist
GS07	22,865,424	25,094,868	Administrative officer
GS08	20,234,904	22,207,812	Psychologist
GS09	17,906,976	19,652,916	Senior registry officer
GS10	15,846,888	17,391,984	Personal secretary
GS11	14,023,800	15,345,876	Assistant accountant
GS12	12,457,848	13,632,252	Cashier
GS13	11,066,760	12,110,040	Typist
GS14	9,831,000	10,757,856	Registry clerk
GS15	8,651,544	9,467,184	Head office orderly

Source: PSMD Circulars B.4 and B.5 of 2007.

Table 3.5   Medical Salary Scale as of April 1, 2007

Scale	Minimum salary (K)	Maximum salary (K)	Example
MS01	54,252,384	56,120,280	Chief nursing officer
MS02	47,714,772	51,450,564	Principal physiotherapist
MS03	42,273,300	44,239,524	Senior nursing officer
MS04	40,184,220	41,806,356	Principal anesthesiologist
MS05	25,495,068	26,871,420	Principal clinical officer
MS06	23,430,564	24,806,916	Public health nurse
MS07	19,168,896	19,989,696	Registered midwife
MS08	15,893,436	16,384,980	Dental therapist
MS09	15,308,508	15,564,108	Pharmacy technician
MS10	14,270,904	14,746,536	Pharmacy dispenser
MS11	12,969,456	13,435,680	Dental attendant

Source: PSMD Circular B.5 of 2007.

Table 3.6   Medical Doctors Salary Scale as of April 1, 2007

Scale	Minimum salary (K)	Maximum salary (K)	Example
MDS01	78,713,508	84,218,868	Director
MDS02	61,279,860	67,178,460	District medical officer
MDS03	54,252,384	56,120,280	Clinical care specialist
MDS04	52,595,856	53,742,816	Senior resident medical officer
MDS05	42,764,856	44,239,524	Pharmacist

Source: PSMD Circular B.4 of 2007.

of location. Allowances that pertain to health workers are shown in table 3.7. These allowances often represent a high proportion of pretax remuneration, as illustrated in table 3.7,[17] where allowances account for 39 percent[18] of a doctor's total remuneration and 21 percent of a lab technician's. For the medical doctor, the on-call allowance (not available to other health professionals) makes the biggest difference in total remuneration compared with the remuneration of other health workers and civil servants.

Allowances are captured as "other emoluments" and are not part of the personnel emoluments from the Ministry of Finance and Planning because they are specific to the health sector and are not paid out consistently. For example, the on-call allowance depends on the number of times the doctor was on call, which is determined retrospectively. Some allowances are donor financed. For example, the Zambia Health Worker Retention Scheme (ZHWRS) is currently available only to a limited number of doctors in rural districts. In 2005, the allowances under this scheme amounted to about US$600 to US$700 per doctor. The ZHWRS is currently being expanded to include nurses and other health workers. Table 3.7 shows the monthly salary for selected cadres of health workers.

There are significant differences in health worker salaries between the private and the public sectors. An HIV/AIDS workforce study report referenced in the HRH strategy stated that the salaries of doctors in the private sector were three times those of government workers. For midwives, those in the private sector earned one-third more than their government counterparts. In addition, laboratory technicians in the private sector were paid three times more than their government counterparts.

Promotion. Promotion in the health sector depends on whether a vacancy is available and whether a recommendation has been made to fill

Table 3.7 Composite Monthly Pay before Tax of Sample of Health Professionals, 2005

Cadre	Gross monthly salary (K)	Recruitment and retention (K)	Commuted overtime (K)	Commuted night duty (K)	Uniform upkeep (K)	Housing allowance (K)	On-call allowance (K)	Grand total (K)	Grand total (US$)	Allowance as share of total (%)
Doctor	3,778,438	755,688	n.a.	n.a.	n.a.	500,000	1,200,000	6,234,126	1,453	39
Pharmacist	3,072,188	614,438	n.a.	n.a.	35,000	400,000	n.a.	4,121,626	960	25
Laboratory scientist	2,687,500	537,500	n.a.	n.a.	35,000	400,000	n.a.	3,660,000	853	27
Tutor	2,429,500	485,900	n.a.	n.a.	35,000	450,000	n.a.	3,400,400	792	29
Senior nurse and paramedic	1,683,230	336,646	40,000	30,000	35,000	450,000	n.a.	2,574,876	600	35
Nurse	1,141,770	n.a.	40,000	30,000	35,000	250,000	n.a.	1,496,770	349	24
Midwife	1,141,770	n.a.	40,000	30,000	35,000	250,000	n.a.	1,496,770	349	24
Clinical officer	1,141,770	n.a.	40,000	30,000	35,000	250,000	n.a.	1,496,770	349	24
Laboratory technologist	1,141,770	n.a.	40,000	30,000	35,000	250,000	n.a.	1,496,770	349	24
Pharmacy technician	1,141,770	n.a.	n.a.	n.a.	35,000	250,000	n.a.	1,426,770	332	20
Laboratory technician	981,354	n.a.	40,000	30,000	35,000	150,000	n.a.	1,236,354	288	21

Source: Zambia Ministry of Health 2005.
Note: n.a. = not applicable. Exchange rate: US$1 = K 4,292 (October 2005).

it. In practice, the supervisor's recommendation for promotion goes to the Human Resource Department of the MOH, which reviews the request and forwards it to the PSMD, which then passes it on to the PSC for approval. After approval, the PSC sends it back down the same path. This process is also plagued by delays.

Termination and sanctioning. According to the government's policy, termination of an established officer may occur at any time by giving the officer three months' notice in writing, exclusive of leave, or by paying the officer three months' salary in lieu of notice.

Disciplinary issues are the responsibility of the employer through district or hospital discipline committees as well as through professional bodies. In the case of nurses, this body is the General Nursing Council, which has the power to strike people off the register for professional misconduct.[19] In practice, minor problems are dealt with in house or locally. Issues adjudged to be severe are referred to higher authorities. In a 2006 Public Expenditure Tracking Survey of health facilities, of a total of 380 staff members who left health facilities, 8 percent were either dismissed or suspended. In another study, in 2005, 12 percent of all attrition among health workers was due to dismissal (Chitah 2005).

Unexplained absenteeism is also a concern in Zambia (see table 3.8). Absenteeism may be caused by a number of reasons, including moonlighting (that is, by public sector doctors who also practice privately). No well-developed system exists for reporting and verifying absenteeism.

Key Messages

From 2000 to 2003, Zambia experienced a sharp increase in the public sector wage bill, growing from 5.3 percent of GDP to 8.0 percent of GDP. In consultation with the IMF, the government of Zambia put into place a hiring freeze to try to control this growth and keep this ratio

Table 3.8   Attendance at Facility of Employment

Cadre	Rural (%)	Urban (%)	Total or average (%)
Doctors (all)	78	47	55
Nurses and midwives (registered or enrolled)	82	71	77
Health-specific health worker total	84	69	77

Source: Herbst and Gijsbrechts 2007.

below 8 percent of GDP. These efforts have been successful, and the public sector wage bill has remained at or below 8 percent of GDP since 2004.

The health sector was explicitly exempted from the overall public sector hiring freeze; however, MOH data show that this exemption was not necessarily honored. The CBOH and health boards were still in place during this time and therefore were able to continue recruitment through their operational grants budget. Although this allowed more money to go toward salaries, it was at the expense of providing necessary health services.

Actual salaries paid to health workers are not always captured under the personnel emoluments line item of the budget. Under the CBOH system, health boards and other grant-aided institutions were able to pay salaries and other top-ups through their operational grants. These amounts were not included in the wage bill calculations. Although most of the health workers employed under the health boards have now been reintegrated into the MOH and therefore are captured as of 2006 under the wage bill data, those health workers still under certain grant-aided institutions are not yet integrated into the health wage bill.

The government of Zambia is committed to increasing the country's health workforce through additional budgetary allocations. Health has been prioritized within the public sector wage bill, remaining constant at 10 percent of the total since 2004. However, the wage bill is declining as a share of overall health expenditure. This result could be driven in large part by the increase in donor funding for health, which is directed at nonwage expenditures, thus skewing the proportion of health expenditure going to wages.

The capacity of the MOH to implement its wage bill budget is low. This stems from large inefficiencies and an inability to recruit. Without improved public sector management, the ambitious scaling-up goals will be difficult to achieve.

The public sector reforms in the health sector—in particular, the delinkage of the provider function from the purchasing function—were incomplete, creating confusion and therefore limiting success. To restore control over human resource management in the health sector, the MOH (in consultation with the government) abolished the boards of health and reverted to the civil service structure under the MOH for all health workers.

Inefficiencies exist in the health sector that constrain the ability to scale up the workforce. Despite additional resources being made available, the sector was unable to fully fill funded posts within the budget cycle. A tension therefore exists between the service delivery need to get staff members in posts as soon as possible and the need to control costs, both by ensuring that the public service does not revert to uncontrolled hiring or abuse of the payroll and by delaying legitimate recruitment to save funds.

The highly centralized nature of hiring processes has led to unresponsive to human resource needs. It has also resulted in a less efficient process and the inability of the MOH to fill funded posts. Much of the paperwork could be performed more rapidly with the use of standard pro formas and word-processing functions of computers.

The delinkage of the health boards from the MOH was never fully carried out. Its implementation was fraught with irregularities, thus creating significant confusion and anxiety among health workers, ultimately leading to abolition of delinkage. The delinking process, however, provided the MOH an avenue for circumventing the wage bill ceilings imposed by the Ministry of Finance and Planning, because the health boards could hire from their grants and other revenue. However, most of the resources were used for recruiting administrative and other support personnel, not clinical workers. Use of these grants for recruiting led to decreased investment in operations and infrastructure.

Decentralization of the recruitment process should be explored. Some benefits were gained from decentralization of recruitment when health boards had more autonomy. These benefits should be studied to see if they could be incorporated into the new system.

Recruitment and retention allowances could be structured to preferentially reward those working in underserved areas. Allowances make up a significant portion of the health workers' salaries. They are not part of the personnel emoluments but are captured as other emoluments. This structure offers an opportunity for increasing remuneration for health workers and for targeting it toward those working in areas of need without upsetting the personnel emoluments wage bill.

Notes

1. Key informant interview with the former permanent secretary, Public Service Management Division, government of Zambia, February 2008.

2. The term *establishment* refers to the approved structure of an organization (including numbers and types of posts); it is not the same as "funded" posts.

3. The genesis of the base figure is unclear, but in the development of the National Human Resources for Health Plan of 2001, it was stated that: "The [Ministry of Health] establishment has not been . . . actively used since 1992" because of the planned delinkage from the public service.

4. Key informant interviews with the permanent secretary, Public Service Management Division, and chief accountant, Ministry of Health, government of Zambia, April 10–11, 2008.

5. Key informant interview with the permanent secretary, Management Development Division, Cabinet Office, government of Zambia, April 7, 2008.

6. Key stakeholders even alleged in interviews that some staff members might have been receiving full salaries from both the CBOH and the Ministry of Health. This allegation could not be verified, given the cumbersome accounting and financial recording systems.

7. However, user fees were abolished in rural areas in 2006, causing serious problems for health facilities relying on these funds to supplement their staffing complement.

8. Four agencies were listed under this category: the CBOH, the Zambian Flying Doctors Scheme, the Nutrition Commission, and the Medical Association of Zambia.

9. Ghost workers may also be created by those who operate the payroll.

10. Each one is individually typed because there is no standard pro forma.

11. It is unclear why this information is not provided on receipt of the letter of appointment, but it may be because many potential employees do not actually act on the letter of appointment and report to the place of posting, particularly if the posting is unfavorable.

12. Approval is rarely refused except in cases where the individual is over the age of 45 and cannot be permanent and pensionable but may be taken on contract.

13. Having given approval for the filling of a vacancy, the PSMD writes to the PSC. The application goes through a series of meetings at the PSC. Then it comes back to the PSMD. The PSMD advises the PSC to advertise, but the line ministry pays for the advertisement. The PSC, working with the PSMD, constitutes a panel with senior management from the line ministry. After the interview, the permanent secretary of the line ministry writes to the permanent secretary of the PSMD, who then makes a formal submission to the PSC. When the PSC is satisfied, it conveys this information back to the PSMD, which then writes to the line ministry, which, in turn, writes a letter of appointment to the individual.

14. Key informant interview with Human Resources Department of the Zambian Ministry of Health, April 10, 2008.

15. The current scheme pays salaries and nonmonetary incentives to health workers who work in designated facilities for a period of three years in 72 MOH priority districts. This scheme is the only recognized retention scheme approved by the cabinet and the PSC.

16. The 2007 Zambia Health Public Expenditure Tracking Survey showed that as many as 50 percent of hospitals have an expatriate doctor, 25 percent have an expatriate nurse, and 14 percent have other expatriate staff members.

17. This table uses the most recent data available giving allowances by cadre. Some are based on Cabinet Office Circular 19 of 2003, and some have subsequently been updated.

18. This proportion will probably have increased following a recent increase in the on-call allowance for doctors, and it is significantly greater for doctors benefiting from the Zambia Health Worker Retention Scheme.

19. The first step before that action would be recommendation for suspension. A major problem is that the General Nursing Council does not have the capacity to respond to complaints. No one has yet been struck off.

References

Chitah, Mukosha. 2005. "Expenditure Ceilings, Human Resources and Health: The Case for Zambia." WEMOS Foundation, Amsterdam.

Goldsbrough, David, and Caesar Cheelo. 2007. "IMF Programs and Health Spending: Case Study of Zambia." Center for Global Development, Washington, DC.

Herbst, Christopher, and Dieter Gijsbrechts. 2007. "Comprehensive and Accurate Information on Health Worker Stock, Profiles, and Distribution (SPD) in Zambia: Analysis of the JICA Data." Presentation prepared for the Human Resources for Health Research Conference, Mulungushi International Conference Center, Lusaka, June 7–8.

IMF (International Monetary Fund). 2004. *Zambia: Poverty Reduction Strategy Paper Progress Report*. IMF Country Report 04/181. Washington, DC: IMF.

———. 2007a. "Zambia: 2006 Article IV Consultation." IMF, Washington, DC.

———. 2007b. "Zambia: Fifth and Sixth Reviews under the Poverty Reduction and Growth Facility Arrangement and Request for Waiver of Nonobservance of Performance Criteria: Staff Report; Press Release on the Executive Board Discussion; and Statement by the Executive Director for Zambia." IMF Country Report 07/209, IMF, Washington, DC.

———. 2008. "Zambia: 2007 Article IV Consultation—Staff Report; Staff Statement; Public Information Notice on the Executive Board Discussion; and Statement by the Executive Director for Zambia." IMF Country Report 08/41, IMF, Washington, DC. http://www.imf.org/external/pubs/ft/scr/2008/cr0841.pdf.

Jeppsson, Anders, and Sam Agatre Okuonzi. 2000. "Vertical or Holistic Decentralization of the Health Sector? Experiences from Zambia and

Uganda." *International Journal of Health Planning and Management* 15: 273–89.

World Bank. 2001. *Zambia Public Expenditure Review—Public Expenditure, Growth, and Poverty: A Synthesis.* Washington, DC: World Bank.

———. 2007. *World Development Indicators 2007.* Washington, DC: World Bank.

———. 2008. *Health Public Expenditure Review 2008.* Washington, DC: World Bank.

Zambia Ministry of Finance and National Planning. 2003. "2004–2006 Medium-Term Expenditure Framework and the 2004 Budget." Green Paper, Zambia Ministry of Finance, Lusaka.

———. 2004. "2005–2007 Medium-Term Expenditure Framework and the 2005 Budget." Green Paper, Zambia Ministry of Finance, Lusaka.

———. 2005. "2006–2008 Medium-Term Expenditure Framework and the 2006 Budget." Green Paper, Zambia Ministry of Finance, Lusaka.

———. 2006. "2007–2009 Medium-Term Expenditure Framework and the 2007 Budget." Green Paper, Zambia Ministry of Finance, Lusaka.

———. 2007. "2008–2010 Medium-Term Expenditure Framework and the 2008 Budget." Green Paper. Zambia Ministry of Finance, Lusaka.

Zambia Ministry of Health. 2005. "National Health Strategic Plan: 2006–2010." Zambia Ministry of Health, Lusaka.

———. 2008. "Ministerial Statement to Parliament on MOH Budget for the Year 2008." Zambia Ministry of Health, Lusaka.

CHAPTER 4

Background Country Study for Rwanda

The Health Wage Bill in Rwanda

The health sector in Rwanda has traditionally had little control over the wage bill budget. This situation looks set to change with the decentralization reforms and the introduction of performance-based grants (PBGs). The reforms have granted the districts more flexibility in the control of the wage bill budget through block grants, and the PBGs could be used to pay salaries and top-ups. Because health workers are employed as part of the civil service, the process begins with the determination of the budget for the public sector wage bill by the Ministry of Finance and Economic Planning (MINECOFIN). Curtailing the public sector wage bill has been critical to creating fiscal space to implement poverty reduction programs. However, striking a balance between macroeconomic targets and the need to increase the health budgets to make health services accessible and also to ensure that Rwanda achieves its Millennium Development Goals is equally important.

Managing the size of the public sector wage bill level is important, given that its mismanagement could cause macroeconomic volatility. High government wages and large employment can push up the wage bill and crowd out other spending. In general, unbridled government wage increases could feed into a general wage-price spiral that undermines competitiveness and could also result in fiscal slippages (Fedelino, Schwartz, and Verhoeven 2006).

There is no explicit wage bill ceiling in the International Monetary Fund (IMF) Poverty Reduction Growth Facility (PRGF) program. However, the government has a budget for the public sector wage bill based on its priorities for spending on wage and nonwage items. The allocation to sectors, which includes line items for wages, is determined by MINECOFIN, following a joint review of sector proposals and is outlined in the Medium-Term Expenditure Framework (MTEF).

Process for Determining the Budget for the Health Wage Bill

In Rwanda, the process for determining the health and education wage bills has gone beyond the traditional percentage increase from the previous year's budget. It has become an interactive process involving the line ministries, MINECOFIN, and development partners, who take into account the needs of all other government sectors and ensure close linkage to the Economic Development and Poverty Reduction Strategy (EDPRS). This yearlong process for determining the budget for the health wage bill is derived from a three-step process (see annex table 4.A.3) that includes the following:

- A joint review process, which involves an analysis of the previous year's budget execution relative to set objectives and a description of orientations for the coming year. It is realized through reports on annual action plans and budget execution and by joint sector reviews.
- A strategic planning period, during which the Ministry of Health (MINISANTE), the Ministry of Education (MINEDUC), and all the other line ministries prepare strategic issues papers, including provisional MTEFs and earmarked transfers. During this period, MINECOFIN prepares the first draft budget framework paper (BFP). The period ends with budget and sector consultations and the finalization of the BFP.
- Budget preparation, which involves the finalization of each ministry's MTEF, including detailed budgets for each sector.

No explicit wage ceilings are mandated by the IMF or included as part of the PRGF. The only major constraint remains the finite nature of the overall budget envelope. In fact, Rwanda has a wage floor that is mandated for spending in priority sectors such as health and education. The determination of the wage bill envelope is an iterative process led by MINECOFIN that takes into account its own revenue projections, the government agreements with the IMF, and the proposals from the sector under consideration. Usually, during the MTEF preparation, the line ministries, on the basis of staffing norms and the number of available candidates, present a request for the funding of a certain number of positions. On receiving the request, MINECOFIN, depending on the total available budget envelope, accepts either the entire request or just part of it. Customarily, the budget envelope is raised by 3 to 5 percent of the previous year's budget (although this is no longer the case in health and education ministries). Between 2005 and 2006, however, the budget envelope jumped by 15 percent. Two important changes have been proffered as the main reasons for this increase:[1] (a) the public sector salary reform that changed the index value[2] from 100 to 250 and (b) an incentives package introduced in 2006.

Contrary to what occurs in some African countries, such as Mali, Niger, Senegal, and Zambia, Rwanda has not included wage ceilings as a conditionality in the PRGFs signed between the government and the IMF since 2003. In fact, the February 2007 PRGF (IMF 2007a) for Rwanda states that priority spending as identified by the Poverty Reduction Strategy Paper, which includes spending on health and education, will increase by at least 1.5 percent of gross domestic product (GDP). For the education sector, additional spending of about 2 percent has already been identified under the Fast Track Initiative (1 percent of GDP) and for so-called contingent spending, which would be allocated in equal proportion to priorities and nonpriorities. Therefore, instead of a ceiling, a floor appears to have been put in place for priority spending. Thus, in theory, no constraints or limits on spending exist for what are considered priority activities. Figures 4.1 and 4.2 show the public sector wage bill for Rwanda (and the entire region) in 2005 as a percentage of GDP and as a percentage of government expenditure.

Nevertheless, the agreement with the IMF to set a limit to the fiscal deficit puts a cap on government expenditures and therefore implicitly limits wages and salaries. When negotiating with MINISANTE and MINEDUC (and with all other line ministries), MINECOFIN sets ceilings on expenditures on the basis of its projected revenues. As a result, although no wage and salary ceilings are explicitly set in the IMF agreement, the ministries negotiate under an expenditure constraint that forces them to limit their wage and salary bills. In fact, MINECOFIN limits the size of the extra workforce that can be hired by those two ministries. (For instance, during the 2008 budget preparation, the number of teachers could be increased by no more than 3 percent.)

Figure 4.1   Public Sector Wage Bill as a Share of GDP, by Country, 2005

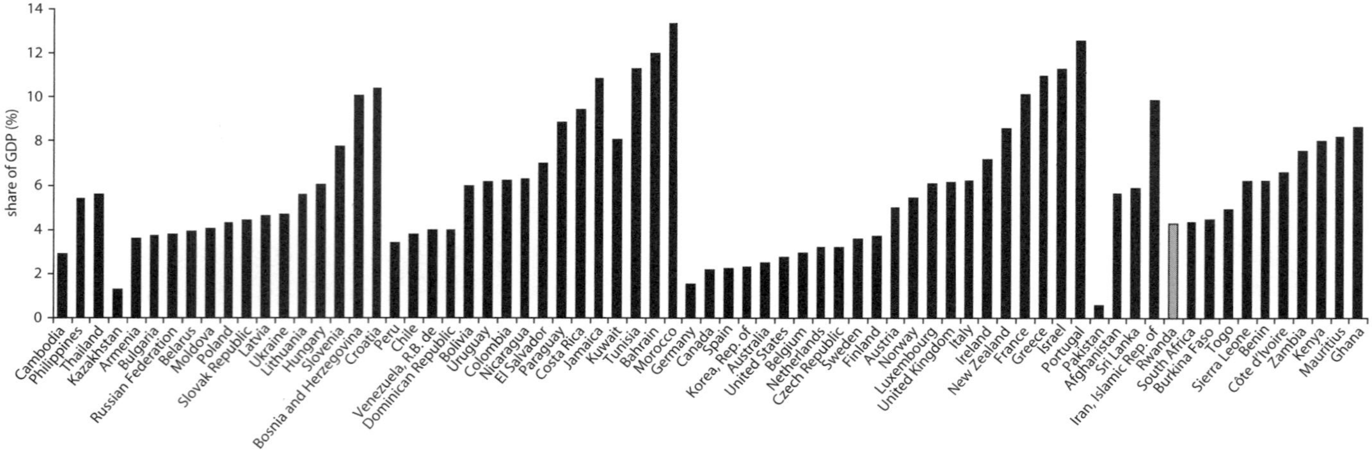

Source: World Bank 2007.

Figure 4.2 Public Sector Wage Bill as a Share of Government Expenditure, by Country, 2005

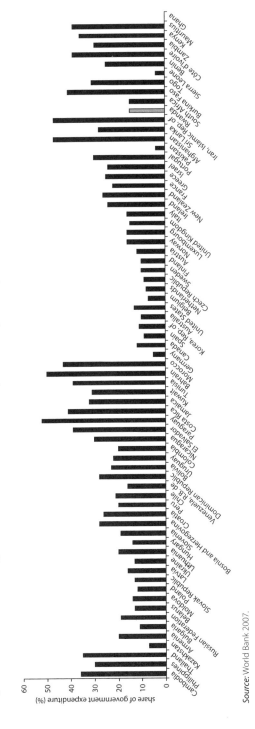

Source: World Bank 2007.

131

Estimates of total expenditure on wages are challenging because of the different levels of government in a decentralized context and different available channels of transfer—some direct, others indirect. In addition, the use of performance-based contracts by design compounds this situation, but it has the desired benefit of tying wages to results.

Expenditures on human resources for health (HRH) occur at different levels in the public system in Rwanda and through several channels that make exactitude challenging (Goldsbrough, Leeming, and Christiansen 2007). As a result, using only the traditional classification of wages and salaries gives a limited view of the real extent of the HRH wage bill. In addition to its usual central administration expenditures, MINISANTE transfers funds to institutions to pay for salaries of health workers, among other things. These transferred funds appear in MINISANTE's budget as subitem transfers.[3] In addition, health workers are also hired at the provincial and district levels—a process accentuated by the decentralization policy being undertaken by the government of Rwanda. These workers are paid both by funds coming through the government and by user fees collected directly by facilities in these districts and provinces.

Funding for HRH has four main sources in Rwanda. The first is the MINISANTE budget for health workers in the central level and for those working in institutions that also receive transfers, such as tertiary centers. The second source is transfers from MINECOFIN to the districts in the form of earmarked funds. The third source is the performance-based grants, some of which may be used to supplement salaries, but which are not necessarily earmarked for that purpose. The fourth source is based on local revenue generated by the facility, such as from user fees, that can be used to hire lower-cadre health workers.

Some of the funds being used to pay health workers' wages and salaries in the districts and provinces do not appear in the government budget. Furthermore, even some of the funds paid by the government do not appear in MINISANTE's budget but are instead included in the budgets of provinces and districts. Therefore, to have a comprehensive picture of what is really spent by the government (from its recurrent budget[4]) on human resources in the health sector, one must take all these three levels into account. This was done to come up with what is referred to in this chapter as *total government recurrent HRH expenditures*.

A very important caveat is that estimates of the total wage bill usually omit payments to staff made from performance-based grants. These grants are not broken down into different components such as salary top-ups. Rather, they appear in the budget section as "Other purchases of goods and services" (subsection "Expenditures not elsewhere classified"[5]).

The PBG was deliberately designed to grant the health facility flexibility in appropriating the grant as deemed necessary, in return for meeting agreed-on targets. However, that flexibility makes separating wage and salary top-ups from other operating expenditures—just by looking at the budget or at budget execution reports—very difficult. This differentiation would require visiting each health facility and collecting the data, which might not always be available. These top-ups allow an increase in the salary of a health worker, sometimes by up to 86 percent (from an index value of 250 to 465[6]).

The PBG provides significant resources that can be used for the payment of salaries and allowances. The amount spent by the government of Rwanda in PBGs is significant; it reached RF 3,439,221,438 of the RF 4,410,522,658 budgeted in 2007 (MINISANTE 2007). If only one-fourth of this amount was spent on wage and salary top-ups (a conservative estimate, according to managers at MINISANTE), this amount would already be sizable. The amount is even larger when donor contributions to the PBGs are taken into consideration. Although PBGs are not included in the analysis, their potential effect on the health wage bill underscores their importance.

Fiscal decentralization has occurred, including in the health sector's wage bill. Direct spending on wages and salaries by MINISANTE is a very small fraction (less than one-tenth) of the total expenditure on wages and salaries (either directly or through transfers) by this ministry (figure 4.3). The wage bill at the central level (MINISANTE) has been declining since 2003 because of cuts in the central-level workforce. In 2006, its share of total HRH expenditures was less than half of what it was in 2003 (declining from 7.7 percent to 3.6 percent).

Wage and salary transfers to public institutions, which used to be the main HRH expenditure items during the period under consideration, are declining. Salaries channeled to the health workforce through provincial and district budgets are rapidly catching up and are expected to constitute the principal item in HRH expenditures for 2007. This development is interesting because wages and salaries that were paid regardless of performance are now partly linked to results because some of those wages are now tied to performance. Most of the funding (close to RF 3.6 billion) is now tied to performance contracts signed by health centers and district hospitals, both because of the desire to improve the quality of health services and because of administrative decentralization reforms that have been under way for the past few years in Rwanda. This trend is also apparent in the education sector (figure 4.4).

Figure 4.3   Distribution of HRH Expenditures as a Share of Total, 2003–07

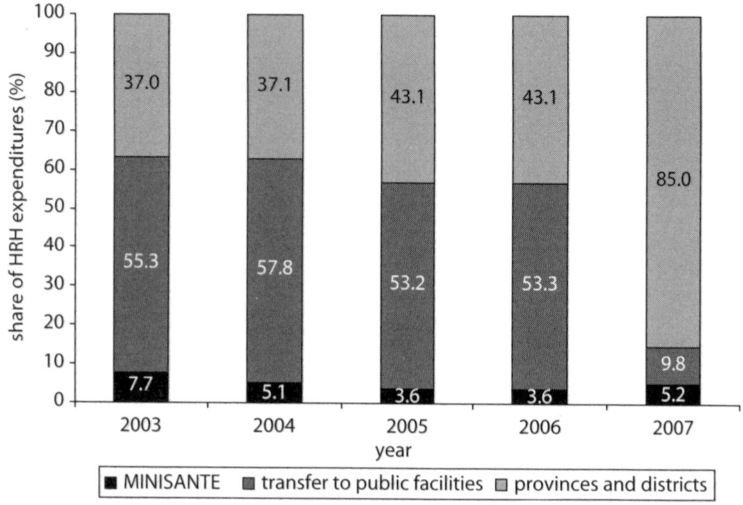

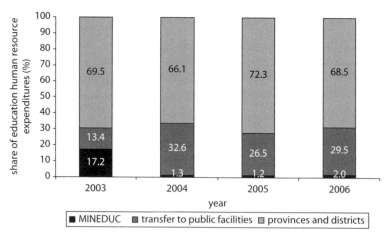

Source: Annex table 4.A.2.

Figure 4.4   Distribution of Education Human Resource Expenditures as a Share of Total, 2003–06

Source: Annex table 4.A.2.

Rwanda is implementing its decentralization process in three phases:

- *Phase 1 (2000–2003)*. Putting in place the necessary policies and legal framework and establishing local government structures, procedures, and systems

- *Phase 2 (2004–2008)*. Empowering local governments and communities to plan, finance, implement, and sustain development through fiscal strengthening and sectoral decentralization, among other activities
- *Phase 3 (2009 onward)*. Consolidating the expected achievements and ensuring that the systems and structures are sustained

In January 2008, wages and salaries for the health sector were decentralized from the central level to the district and facility levels. At the present stage of this decentralization process (phase 2), districts obtain public funding for HRH from three sources: (a) earmarked funds in the form of transfers from MINECOFIN to the provinces for HRH wages and salaries (these are basically delegated funds); (b) HRH motivation funds (for health workers in communities, health centers, and district hospitals); and (c) the PBGs (block transfers that could, among other things, finance HRH).

The decentralization of budgets, along with the flexibility in how the PBGs can be used, has provided districts and facilities much more control over the health wage bill. Facilities can supplement the salary budget from the earmarked funds with funds from the PBGs. These grants make up a significant portion of revenues for facilities and provide considerable scope for increasing the wage bill budget. As a safeguard against using it all for salaries, at least 25 percent of the total PBG has to be committed to nonwage expenditure, such as maintenance, goods, and services (MINISANTE 2008).

Results of the Wage Bill Budgeting Process

The policy priorities of the government of Rwanda are to control spending and to make sure that the wage and salary bill does not get out of control. After cuts in the public workforce brought down the wage bill from 4.8 percent in 2003 to 4.3 percent in 2005, the share of direct wages and salaries (measured according to the IMF definition) in GDP recovered in 2006 to a 4.7 percent level. This share was projected to decline briefly in 2007 before remaining stable at 4.7 percent for the next two years (figure 4.5). This same trend remains when the wage and salary bill is taken relative to total government expenditures (including net lending). The public sector wage bill is projected to decline from 20.0 percent of government expenditure in 2003 to 16.1 percent in 2009 (figure 4.6). This reduction shows a concerted effort by the government of Rwanda to reallocate resources away from wages and salaries and toward other budgetary items.

Figure 4.5   Public Sector Wage Bill and Recurrent Government Human Resource Expenditure as a Share of GDP, 2003–09

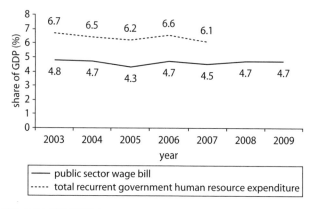

Sources: IMF 2007a, 2007b; MINEDUC 2007.

Note: Data for 2007, 2008, and 2009 are based on budget estimates.

Figure 4.6   Public Sector Wage Bill and Recurrent Government Human Resource Expenditure as a Share of Government Expenditure, 2003–09

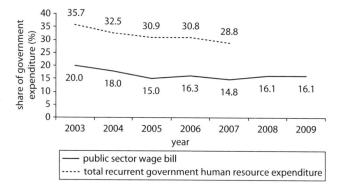

Sources: IMF 2007a, 2007b; MINEDUC 2007.

Note: Data for 2007, 2008, and 2009 are based on budget estimates.

If the more comprehensive measure for total recurrent government HR expenditures (computed from MINECOFIN data) is used, the share of HRH expenditure in GDP, although higher than the noncomprehensive measure presented in the figure 4.5 (remaining at over 6 percent for the period), still shows a relatively stable level, slightly declining from 2003 to 2005 before barely recovering in 2006. However, it is projected to decrease in 2007. When these comprehensive HR expenditure levels are taken relative to recurrent expenditures, the decline becomes more pronounced, with a drop from over 35 percent in 2003 to below 31 percent in 2006 and even lower values (less than 29 percent) projected for 2007. The main message here is that overall recurrent government expenditures on the wage bill, although stable relative to GDP, have declined during this period. The questions now are whether human resources in the health and education sectors have been affected by this decline, whether they have been protected relative to other sectors, and how these two sectors have dealt with the overall decline in the government recurrent wage bill.

The health sector has accounted for an increasing share of both the public sector wage bill and the overall government health expenditures. Figure 4.7 shows this increasing trend of the health wage bill as a share of the public sector wage bill, with health comprising 5.6 percent of the public sector wage bill in 2003 and a projected 9.3 percent by 2007. In light of the overall wage bill cuts, health is taking a larger share of the overall wage bill budget, revealing a clear prioritization of the health wage bill relative to other sectors.

Health expenditure as a proportion of total government expenditure also showed an increasing trend, although it dipped in 2006 after a significant rise in 2005. This trend illustrates some prioritization of health (figure 4.8).

The health wage bill as a proportion of total health expenditure has remained fairly constant from 2003 to 2006, except for the dip in 2005. This is in contrast to the education sector, where the ratio has steadily decreased (figure 4.9). Not too much can be read into this fact because of a virtual delinking of the processes that account for the numerator and

Figure 4.7   Health Wage Bill as a Share of Public Sector Wage Bill, 2003–07

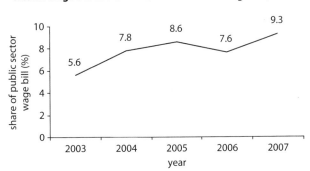

Source: Annex table 4.A.2
Note: Data for 2007 are based on budget estimates.

Figure 4.8   Health Expenditure as a Share of Government Expenditure and Health Wage Bill as a Share of Health Expenditure, 2003–06

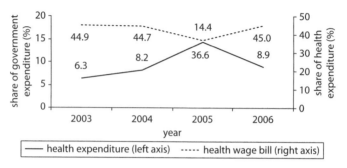

Source: Computed from annex table 4.A.2.

Figure 4.9   Share of Wages in Sector Recurrent Expenditures, 2003–07

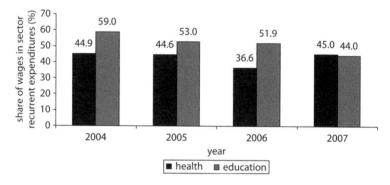

Source: Computed from annex table 4.A.2.

denominator. Budgeting for the health wage bill is largely independent of the budgeting process for nonwage health expenditure.[7] The projections for 2007 show a trend reversal; however, this finding simply reflects the numerator growing at a larger rate than the denominator. Again, the share of health spending devoted to wages is not a strategic decision in the traditional budgeting setup.

Overall, the health sector has been unable to fully execute its ordinary human resource budget over the past few years (2003–06), and the execution rate has varied considerably from year to year (figure 4.10). The performance of MINISANTE has been uneven over this period, with full budget execution occurring only in 2006. At the province and district levels, however, the reverse is true—budgeted amounts have always been totally spent, except in 2006. A sharp reduction in budget execution

Figure 4.10   Health Wage Bill Budget Wage Bill Execution Rate, 2003–06

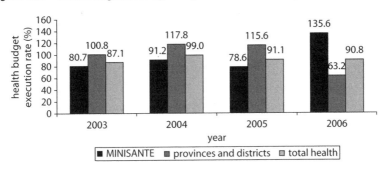

Source: Computed from annex table 4.A.2.

occurred at the local level in 2006. The reason for the contrasting per-
formances at the local level is unclear. Changes in fiduciary arrangements
with the advent of decentralization and limited capacity to manage
increased wage bill budgets at the local level may have contributed.

The trends are completely different for the education sector, where,
except for 2005, the human resource budget has always been totally
spent during the period. MINEDUC always spent all (or more than) its
available budget, and the provinces and districts were generally very stable in executing what was set aside for them in the annual budgets.
Consequently, education shows a budget execution rate of 100 percent or
more (except in 2005), possibly highlighting the improvements in
MINEDUC's management and planning capacity.

Despite data limitations, estimates of government health workers show
an increasing trend between 2003 and 2006. Data on the evolution of the
health workforce has been very difficult to find; hence, renewed efforts
are being made to establish a reliable database to address the large dis-
crepancies between figures collected by different sources (table 4.1).
MINISANTE, MINEDUC, and the Ministry of Public Service and Labour
(MIFOTRA) are all unable to provide precise figures on the number of
health and education workers recruited in the public system or leaving it.
The time series data show that new health workers are being recruited,
which is consistent with the prioritization of health.

Public Sector Employment of Health Workers

Several changes have occurred in civil service employment in the past few
years. In 1999, the staffing was rationalized, reducing the workforce to

Table 4.1   Estimated Size of Publicly Funded Health Workforce in Rwanda, 2003–06

Health workforce	2003	2005	2006
Doctors	204	221	255
Nurses	2,314	4,107	4,344
Other	2,617	1,159	2,392
Total	5,135	5,487	6,991

Sources: For 2003: Furth, Gass, and Kagubare 2005 (but total is said to be 4,889 instead of 5,135); for 2005, MINISANTE 2006a; for 2006, Herbst 2007.

about 8,500 employees from 11,000. Each ministry managed the staff in its sector at the central and decentralized levels.[8] Other reforms in 2003, 2004, and 2005 involved further staff rationalization and decentralization of responsibilities to the districts, with a significant reduction in central-level personnel. The health and education sectors were usually excluded from these reforms.

More recently, the health and education sectors have introduced some reforms. In the health sector, the index value was modified, leading to an increase in human resource expenditures that resulted in a deficit of RF 600 million, according to MINISANTE's Planning Department. To control its budget, MINISANTE decided to cut its staff in February 2007. Five hundred A4-level employees, the least-qualified category of personnel, were dismissed and were given a severance package that was based on their previous salary and experience levels.

Creating Funded Posts in the Health Sector

Two main categories of vacancies occur in the health sector: those for centrally funded positions and those funded from local resources. The former are typically regular civil service positions. Vacancies for these civil service posts are approved during the MTEF process. After MINECOFIN approves the additional wage bill budget for the health sector, vacancies are created and considered approved. For the second category, funding is derived from local resources, such as user fees and other revenue sources. Staff members recruited under this method are usually short-term and contract-based. Nevertheless, the positions for which they are being recruited have to be within the establishment. These workers usually accept remuneration from the district that is often less than the regular wage with the hope of being "regularized" at the next budget cycle.

Recruiting Health Workers in the Public Sector

According to the civil service statutes, recruitment can happen only if a vacant post exists in the organizational structure and if it has been budgeted for. Such a recruitment process to fill public service positions is competitive and follows the usual process of advertising positions, receiving applications, proceeding to a test (or *concours*), and selecting the best candidate (see rules in the civil service statutes). However, for certain positions in MINISANTE, such as doctors and other A0- and A1-level health workers, the supply of qualified workers is so low that all available workers are automatically recruited and offered positions.

Since the beginning of 2008, recruitment procedures have changed with the introduction of a decentralized budget management process. Recruitment is carried out at two levels, depending on staff category. For doctors and other A0- and A1-level personnel, the health facility is required to send a request to the minister of health, who then approves the request (depending on available vacancies in the facility) before hiring can take place. For staff at the A2-level and below, the health facility can recruit and hire directly, provided that there is a vacancy in the health facility. The new procedures do not allow recruiting if MINISANTE has not already identified a vacancy.

The centrally determined budget envelope for hiring regular health workers constitutes a fiscal space constraint, which the local authorities may circumvent by employing workers at levels A2 and below on a contractual basis. According to human resource officers at MINISANTE, the entire recruitment process takes an average of 70 days from the time a position is posted to the time the new hire can start working. In essence, the local level has the authority to select, test candidates, and hire staff members up to the A2 level. However, the budget envelope for the wage bill is fixed at the central level. Therefore, the fiscal space for hiring health workers at the local level on civil service contracts is not within the control of the local authority. This constraint is circumvented, however, because the local authority can employ health workers on non–civil service contracts, funding the position through user fees and other revenue sources.

Once recruited and appointed, the health or education staff member (and indeed any civil servant) goes through the hiring process, which starts with an oath. The oath-taking ceremony is followed by a six-month probation period at the end of which the staff member is either confirmed or dismissed.

Terms of Work in the Public Sector

Terms of work include tenure, remuneration, promotion and transfers, and termination and sanctions.

Tenure. In Rwanda, public sector employment in both the health and education sectors is managed by two sets of regulations—the Civil Service Commission Regulations and the *Code du Travail*. The Civil Service Commission Regulations apply to all employees hired on a regular basis by the government, whereas the *Code du Travail* regulates employees hired by the government on a contractual basis. In MINISANTE, a sub-policy for human resources has been developed but is still under review and is not yet available as a legal document. According to the *Human Resources for Health Strategic Plan 2006–2010* (MINISANTE 2006a), the cabinet has authorized the formulation of specific statutes to govern health professionals.

Three types of employees appear in the Finance Law (table 4.2). Statutory employees are regular civil servants who are not limited in their tenure of service and may work until retirement. These employees are governed by the civil service statutes. For the nonstatutory employee or the contractual employee, however, the length of work is limited, and they both are on contracts either with the central government or with the health facilities. Funding could come straight from MINECOFIN, MINISANTE (directly or through transfers), the facility itself, a donor, or a nongovernmental organization. Some nonstatutory employees are assimilated as statutory and, as such, are under the civil service statutes, whereas all other contractual employees are governed by the Labour Code.

This system has changed. Currently, all health workers are considered staff of the government. With the introduction of PBGs, the health providers are to be contracted and managed by health facilities at the local level, which will have the authority to hire and fire on the basis of workers' performance and the needs of the health facility, in line with the national HRH strategy. In practice, however, this structure may be

Table 4.2   Types of Contracts in the Civil Service

Type of contract	Benefits	Length of contract
Statutory (includes medical civilian personnel)	Defined by the civil service statutes	Not limited; guaranteed job and subject is "pensionable"
Nonstatutory (deputies, representatives, expatriate personnel, senators, commissioners)		Limited to position tenure length or by a contract
Contractual (includes teachers)	Negotiable and governed by the Labour Code	Limited duration according to contract

Sources: Adapted from the Finance Law and from the civil service statutes of Rwanda.

difficult to enforce for the following reasons. First, the shortage of certain cadres of health workers, such as doctors, makes finding replacements for fired employees difficult. Second, hiring certain cadres, such as doctors, requires a lengthy process and the approval of MINISANTE. Hiring is easier for lower-cadre staff. Third, no standardized performance-based assessment tools are available; thus, evaluation is at the discretion of the facilities, which have varying capacity to manage performance.

Therefore, with respect to how workers are paid and their governing jurisdictions, the following types of workers exist:

- *Workers at the central level.* These workers include (a) MINISANTE's own staff and (b) the staffs of tertiary facilities under the jurisdiction of MINISANTE. These facilities receive direct transfers from MINISANTE.
- *Workers at the local level (provinces and districts).* These workers are under the jurisdiction of the districts and the health facilities, as previously explained, and include (a) provincial and district office staff members and (b) health professionals at the facilities. These facilities receive most of their funding directly from MINECOFIN through the district's budget line. In addition, they receive PBGs from MINISANTE and also from MINECOFIN that can be used for salary top-ups or other operating expenditures.

In addition, MINISANTE has not yet fully developed accreditation systems for health professionals or facilities, although forthcoming changes in the training program for medical doctors include a licensing mechanism. Although required by statute, no standardized performance appraisals are systematically performed for health workers throughout the system (MINISANTE 2006a). With the introduction of PBGs, however, the facilities are expected to set performance targets for the health workers, attached to incentives—sometimes financial—against which some of the grants may be applied.

Remuneration. Salaries are now attached to specific positions instead of to the employee. This system is intended to reduce variability in wages among employees occupying posts of the same level. The basic parameter on which salaries are based has been recently modified by the civil service reform. Salaries are no longer based on the diploma carried by the person who occupies a position but instead on the position occupied. Hence, every position has to be evaluated and classified in terms of a set of criteria, and everyone who holds that position should have the same base salary.

Two elements are used to determine the salary: an index value (that is, a multiplier) and the actual index. For health staff members in districts, the index value, which was 100, was changed to 250 in the last reform. For health staff members in reference hospitals, this index value was increased to 600 from its initial value of 100. Every post is assigned an index, and the higher the post, the higher the index. The differences in salaries between two people holding the same position is then based on the allowances they receive.

In the health sector, allowances have been used historically to circumvent the base salaries in the civil service. In the health sector, new housing allowances and loans that target doctors who fulfill a set of criteria have been introduced. Before the reform, these allowances and premiums were the main instruments used to circumvent the low level of base salaries. The main allowances used in the civil service system were the housing allowance and the transport allowance. In addition to the housing allowance, managers at MINISANTE's Planning Department explained that the ministry has put in place plans to facilitate housing loans for doctors. This benefit will apply mostly to doctors who fulfill the following criteria: they work in rural areas, they have more than four years of service in the public sector, and they do not already own a house. The benefit will also extend to surgeons and anesthetists in urban areas (who are in short supply).[9]

Before the reform, a "premium" was also added to the total remuneration of the employee. The value of this premium could vary widely and often caused major distortions in pay levels between people occupying equivalent positions. For instance, an administrator in the Ministry of Justice could receive a premium that would make his total remuneration several times higher than that of another administrator at the same level and with similar qualifications and experience but who happened to work in a different sector with a lower premium. To harmonize salaries, the reform eliminated this premium, and only the housing and transport allowances have been retained. MINISANTE has stated its intention to introduce differentials that are based on location, but at present, allowances are the same for individuals occupying the same position, no matter where the job is located.

The share of allowances as a proportion of total remuneration has decreased over the years both at the central level and in the health sector as a whole. The reverse has been the case in the education sector. This situation gives the health sector less room for using allowances to reward desired health worker behaviors and trends, such as willingness to work in remote locations.

Although the share of total remuneration accounted for by salaries and allowances is quite high for both sectors and both at central level and in provinces and districts, health and education show opposite trends overall (figures 4.11 and 4.12).

The share of allowances relative to total remuneration has decreased over time in the health sector, whereas in the education sector, it has generally increased. At global levels, allowances represent a higher share of the total human resource expenditures in the education sector than they do in health (31.1 percent in education compared with 21.0 percent in health).

Promotions and transfers. Staff promotions are supposed to be based on performance evaluations. In practice, however, this requirement is not strictly adhered to, perhaps because of capacity constraints and the lack

Figure 4.11   Components of the Health Wage Bill, 2003–06

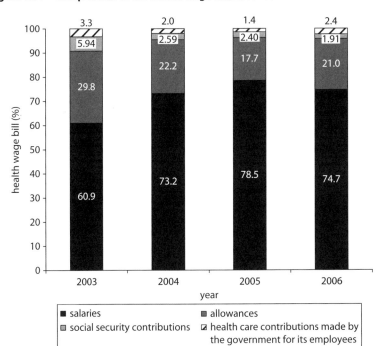

Source: Computed from annex table 4.A.2.

Figure 4.12   Components of the Education Wage Bill, 2003–06

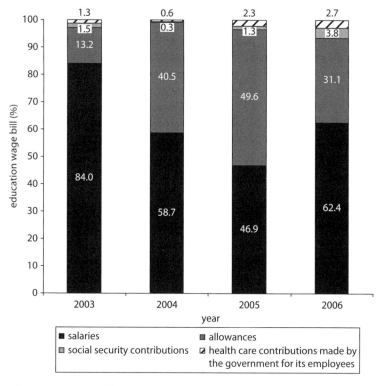

Source: Computed from annex table 4.A.2.

of an effective performance evaluation mechanism. Promotions for employees in both sectors follow the rules set forth in the civil service statutes. Promotion is contingent on an annual evaluation by the immediate superior or supervisor. This evaluation is the basis for determining whether the employee will be promoted and receive a salary increase. In practice, however, promotion rules reportedly are not always followed, and people can stay at the same level for quite a long time.

Health workers are not equitably distributed, with most working in urban areas. The incentive structures and the system of transfers and automatic payments have not allowed this imbalance to be corrected. About 83 percent of health professionals are posted in the urban areas (MINISANTE 2006a). Reasons include the difference in earning potential and access to opportunities and social services, such as schools. Incentive packages for doctors posted to rural areas have been introduced but have not been sufficient to address the issue. Not surprisingly, the rural areas suffer from acute shortages of health workers.

One issue that makes this situation worse is the system of staff transfers. Two factors come to light. The first is the practice by which MIFOTRA makes automatic payments to the health professional, regardless of where he or she works; hence, the money follows the health worker instead of the position. Second is the lack of effective oversight by MINISANTE over the transfers, because the law allows provincial and district authorities to transfer staff members within a province or a district without prior approval from MINISANTE. This situation makes human resource planning in this sector difficult because the movement of staff is difficult to follow. One health center could be overstaffed whereas another could be understaffed. At the same time, the health center from which the transferred staff members came could face a shortage if it is unable to attract people to replace departing personnel.

By stopping automatic payments to individuals and basing payments on approved posts in facilities, the government has been able to improve its data on the distribution of health workers and ensure that facilities either are staffed or have resources to hire staff. Since January 2008, each health center has the same posts, but staff management has been shifted directly to the health facilities, thereby removing the automatic nature of salary payments made by MIFOTRA and involving the districts in the payment chain. Just as the civil service statutes state that "recruitment is possible only if there is a vacant post in the organizational structure and if included in the budget," transfers are now possible only if the person being transferred would be occupying elsewhere the same post he or she is leaving. The salary does not follow the employee anymore, but rather is tied to the post, and this salary is directly managed by the health facility. Thus, if an employee left his or her position for any reason, a funded vacant position would be available in that health facility, and it would merely have to recruit someone else to fill that position. The employee who left his or her job would have to find a health facility where a funded vacancy existed for the same position he or she left.

Another major problem confronting both the health and education sectors that was induced by staff transfers to the districts as part of the decentralization process is how those decentralization policies affected the capacity of the central ministry to manage the sector. Following decentralization of functions and posts, central levels in both sectors have been left with a minimal staff to manage their responsibilities (35 people for health and 40 for education). As noted in the education public expenditure review (MINEDUC 2007), this structure overloads staff and hinders a department's work. But finding suitable staff members to fill available posts has also been difficult. The health sector has found the proper response by further decentralizing some of its management responsibilities since January 2008 and giving the sole responsibility of district staff management to district health facilities. This structure allows the central staff to focus on policies, rules and regulations, and planning. The drawback will be the learning curve that health facilities will have to go through before being fully able to master the management tools needed for their new tasks.

Linked to promotions and transfers is postgraduate training. The government of Rwanda has put in place policies to ensure that, as much as possible, most training is carried out in the country. Health workers going out of the country for training are required to sign an agreement or bond to return to the country and work for MINISANTE for at least three years. In addition, priority for postgraduate training will be given to candidates who have spent at least two years in public service at the district level. Implementation of the bond arrangement has not been perfect. Some reports indicate that sometimes health workers do not return or that they leave government service before fulfilling the three-year requirement. Sanctions for defaulters are unclear and may not be implemented.

Termination and sanctions. According to the civil service statutes, a government worker who has breached employment obligations can be subjected to two types of disciplinary sanctions: first- or second-degree sanctions. First-degree sanctions can be imposed by the competent authority, such as the management of the health facility, whereas second-degree sanctions require consultations with the Civil Service Commission. The actual practice is unclear, as is the detailed nature of these sanctions. No performance evaluations are consistently performed, and it is hoped that the professional associations will contribute to performing them.

Donor Funding of Health and Education Workers' Salaries

Donor financing plays a significant role in the economic development of Rwanda, accounting for a significant contribution to the Economic Development and Poverty Reduction Strategy. Donors are major players in the economic development of Rwanda and are expected to remain so. Their total contribution to the EDPRS for 2008 to 2012 (MINECOFIN 2007) is expected to reach 39.66 percent.[10] Budgetary commitments to the EDPRS are expected to cover at least 24.80 percent of the total costs of that strategy, and project grants and loans are estimated to cover 14.86 percent. Donor involvement can be tracked by looking at the development budget, where donors' funding intentions are usually shown, and also by taking into account the size of the off-budget amounts injected by some donors through projects and programs—for instance the U.S. Agency for International Development (USAID) through the U.S. President's Emergency Plan for AIDS Relief (PEPFAR) project (PEPFAR 2007). Tracking what is really spent is a difficult exercise that is done by the Central Public Investments and External Finance Bureau (CEPEX), among others.[11] Even with such tracking, however, finding what is allocated to human resource payments is a daunting task.

The health and education sectors have greatly benefited from donor funding in recent years. In the health sector, pledged amounts have increased over the years (see table 4.3). The share of the development budget spent on human resources hired in donor-funded projects or programs does not appear explicitly in available documents.[12]

The high level of development expenditure in 2006 was due to an unexpected increase in grants provided by the Global Fund to Fight AIDS, Tuberculosis, and Malaria (GFATM), the Belgian government, and the International Development Association (an increase of RF 18.3 billion, RF 5 billion, and RF 3 billion, respectively, over what was earmarked in the development budget). In addition, PEPFAR funding almost doubled between 2004 and 2006 (see PEPFAR 2007). In fact, at approximately RF 40 billion, PEPFAR funding for 2006 accounted for about two-thirds of total spending in the health sector (see table 4.3).

Table 4.3   Selected Health Sector Funding Sources, 2004–06

Source	Amount (RF million)		
	2004	2005	2006
PEPFAR funding to Rwanda[a]	21,583	32,950	39,656
Total health recurrent expenditures	11,734	14,318	18,018
Total health expenditures	18,280	29,471	62,291

Sources: PEPFAR 2007; MINECOFIN database.
a. The actual figures are US$39,240,985, US$59,909,487, and US$72,102,434, respectively, for 2004 to 2006, converted at a rate of US$1 = RF 550.

These aid amounts put tremendous pressure on the resources in MIN-ISANTE for effectively managing these funds and balancing this activity with other priorities of the health sector. The exact effect of donor financing on the health sector is yet to be studied.

In the health sector, donor funding is accounted for mostly by targeted financing for specific diseases. In contrast, donor funding in the education sector is much more coordinated, and most funds are channeled through the sector budget. A donor coordination mechanism has been created under the leadership of the U.K. Department for International Development, the main funding agency in the education sector. As a result, labor market distortion is minimized in this sector because major donors have channeled most of their funding through general or sector budget support. By doing so, they have aligned their funding with the national education strategy, and their actions and funding are guided by the government's aid policy, the education memorandum of understanding, and the Budget Law. Thus, spending on human resources by donors is fully integrated into the national budget.

With the introduction of the new policy for financing HRH using the national pay scale, the impact of wage distortions is expected to be mitigated. In the health sector, the use of donor funds has been shifted for financing HRH. MINISANTE has a new human resource policy of collaborating with development partners and harmonizing the framework for compensation packages of health professionals. The objective is to ensure that donors in the health sector use the national pay scale for health workers to minimize distortions in the distribution of health workers and to avert an exodus of health workers from the public sector to donor projects because of the significant pay differentials. In light of this concern, donors such as the GFATM have begun to apply national pay scales and to fully integrate staff members within the health system at large. How widely this new policy has been implemented by various donors is not clear.

Key Messages

The overarching message is that, despite the relative contraction of the public sector wage bill, Rwanda has not only protected the health sector, but also succeeded through decentralization and the introduction of performance-based financing in linking salaries to performance in the health sector.

Within a shrinking public sector wage bill, the health sector has been effectively protected. The share of the public sector wage bill devoted to health has increased substantially. The limited evidence suggests that recruitment has continued in the health sector, resulting in increased staffing levels.

Within the health sector, however, recurrent wage bill expenditure has declined relative to nonwage health expenditures. This trend reflects the separation of the budgeting process for the wage bill from that of nonwage health expenditure. MINISANTE does not have full authority over how much to allocate to wages and how much to allocate to nonwage expenditure from a given health budget.

The decentralization of budgets, along with the implementation of the performance-based grants scheme, has had positive effects. First, it has increased the resource envelope available for hiring health workers because of the flexibility in how PBGs can be used. Second, it has linked payments to health workers with performance by linking the salary top-up amounts paid out of the grants to service delivery results. The performance-based financing scheme has allowed an alignment of financial resources with results, which has the potential to link payments to health workers with performance.

Public sector management capacity could be strengthened. First, a disconnect exists between the process for determining the health wage bill (which is outside MINISANTE's control) and that for nonwage expenditure (which is within MINISANTE's control). This situation makes planning human resources for health difficult. Second, MINISANTE could improve efficiency of wage bill spending by better allocation and management of its staff. In fact, several promising reforms are already under way.

The health wage bill budget execution rate has not been satisfactory. This shows the need for better management and planning capacity. This situation contrasts with the education sector, where the budget has always been fully executed, perhaps reflecting a difference in management and planning capacity.

Vacancies are created in the health sector during the MTEF process; hence, the approval of funded positions is not entirely within the control of the health sector but can be influenced during the MTEF negotiation process. However, with the decentralization reforms, districts and district-level facilities have more autonomy in hiring workers within their establishment.

Lower-cadre workers (A1, A2) can be hired directly by the health facility on a contract, and contractual arrangements for service provision can also be handled by the facilities. This method is often used to circumvent fiscal space constraints. However, it requires significant capacity at health facility level, and whether such capacity is widespread remains unclear.

Recently, salaries have been attached to specific positions instead of the employee. This reduces variability in wages among employees occupying posts of the same level. In addition, automatic payments to staff members irrespective of where they move has been discontinued to reduce the probability of some hospitals disproportionately having more funded positions than others because of staff movement.

The share of allowances as a proportion of the total remuneration has decreased over the years. This is true both at the central level and at the local level and gives the health sector less room to use allowances to reward desired health worker behaviors, including willingness to work in remote locations. The PBGs, however, make this issue less of a concern because they clearly have the potential to fill this role.

Performance evaluation and monitoring are not systematically carried out, making the implementation of sanctions ad hoc and challenging.

Donor funding in the health sector is significant and could be better coordinated. The actual contribution to HRH is difficult to accurately determine, but rough estimates show it to be significant and able to cause distortions. This problem is being addressed through cooperation with donor agencies, which are adopting the national pay scale in remuneration of health workers. The education sector adopts a more harmonized approach, which emphasizes alignment of spending with national strategy and, in some cases, the budget.

Annex

Annex Table 4.A.1   Budget Items Used to Compute Government Recurrent HRH Expenditures

	Budget item	
	Included	Not included
Wages and salaries		
Central level	• D111: Nonstatutory workers	
	• D112: Statutory workers	
	• D113: Contractual workers	
	• D114: Military and police personnel	
Exceptional expenditures	• D171: Wages and salaries	
Subsidies to public institutions	• D331: Wages and salaries	• D341: Transfers to nonprofit private institutions

Annex Table 4.A.1   Budget Items Used to Compute Government Recurrent HRH Expenditures (*Continued*)

	Budget item	
	Included	*Not included*
Other purchases of goods and services (other expenditures not elsewhere classified)		• D16918: Conditional support to health centers • D16921: Conditional support to health district centers • D16922: Conditional support to district hospitals • D16928: Conditional support to reference hospitals
Allowances		
Central level	• D116: Allowances and other benefits	
Exceptional expenditures	• D172: Allowances and other benefits	
Subsidies to public institutions	• D332: Allowances and other benefits	
Other goods and services expenditures for districts	• D33884: Health centers personnel motivation • D33385: Community contractual approach • D33892: District hospital personnel motivation	
Social contributions		
Central level	• D121: Employer contribution to CSS • D122: Contribution to retirement pensions and provident fund • D123: Employer contribution to health care	
Exceptional expenditures	• D173: Employer contribution to CSS • D174: Employer contribution to health care	
Subsidies to public institutions	• D333: Subscription to CSS • D334: Employer contribution to health care	

Source: Government of Rwanda Finance Laws.
Note: Transfers to nonprofit private institutions were not included because salaries could not be separated from other functioning expenditures. For provinces and districts, wages and salaries for the health sector include gender and social health promotion, while for the education sector, sociocultural development is included. These amounts tend to overstate the actual spending in the two sectors.

Annex Table 4.A.2 Database Used for Calculations, 2003–07

	2003		2004		2005		2006		2007
	Actual	Budget	Actual	Budget	Actual	Budget	Actual	Budget	Budget
Population (million)	8.9		9.1		9.2		9.3		9.4
GDP (RF million)	905,297.3		1,054,272.0		1,197,205.0		1,316,100.0		1,491,800.0
GDP per capita (RF million)	101,718.8		115,854.1		130,131.0		141,516.1		158,702.1
Total government expenditure, including capital (local + donor funded) (RF million)			288,907.9	334,545.2	360,881.0	368,283.9	433,230.5	404,738.2	506,745.1
Total government expenditure, including locally funded capital (RF million)							316,502.5	323,005.8	
Total recurrent government expenditure (RF million)	169,750.1		208,957.4	247,773.5	240,271.2	262,463.3	281,539.8	293,365.0	324,875.6
Total health expenditure, including capital (local + donor funded) (RF million)			18,280.0	19,666.3	29,470.6	32,086.3	62,290.5	36,632.3	44,951.0
Total health expenditure, including locally funded capital (RF million)				12,443.9		16,730.1	19,073.4	19,299.8	20,390.0
Total recurrent health expenditure (MINISANTE + decentralization) (RF million)			11,733.7	12,193.7	14,318.1	15,176.6	18,017.9	18,444.8	19,267.0

Total recurrent health expenditure (MINISANTE only) (RF million)		7,747.5	8,212.7	9,673.6	10,536.4	11,988.8	11,266.7	14,006.9
Total education expenditure, including capital (local + donor funded) (RF million)		43,531.6	48,515.3	55,318.6	54,019.3	67,328.3	65,942.2	84,819.9
Total education expenditure, including locally funded capital (RF million)			40,423.1		48,737.9	60,919.3	59,447.7	78,038.9
Total recurrent education expenditure (MINEDUC + decentralization) (RF million)		39,298.0	39,663.6	45,352.6	45,746.5	56,758.2	55,940.1	71,958.9
Total recurrent education expenditure (MINEDUC only) (RF million)		21,186.3	20,417.1	25,902.3	25,484.8	34,126.2	33,208.8	34,649.4
Total government payments to human resources (RF million)	60,646.0	60,836.6	68,003.0	66,596.3	74,192.0	75,629.8	86,835.0	86,362.0	93,561.8
Salaries (RF million)	45,869.0	44,509.0	49,138.0	45,888.0	51,195.0	50,215.0	64,735.0	63,584.0	67,503.6
Allowances (RF million)	11,995.0	13,174.0	14,708.0	16,960.0	18,373.0	20,124.0	15,744.0	16,167.0	17,960.4
Social security contributions (RF million)	1,446.0	1,669.0	1,889.0	1,810.0	2,008.0	2,315.0	2,631.0	2,869.0	2,642.7
Health care contributions made by the government for its employees (RF million)	1,336.0	1,485.0	2,268.0	1,938.0	2,615.0	2,976.0	3,725.0	3,743.0	5,455.2

(continued)

Annex Table 4.A.2   Database Used for Calculations, 2003-07 (Continued)

	2003 Actual	2003 Budget	2004 Actual	2004 Budget	2005 Actual	2005 Budget	2006 Actual	2006 Budget	2007 Budget
Total central government wage bill, including wage transfers (RF million)			48,455.9		51,149.9		62,194.5	61,743.7	68,679.2
Total public payments to HRH (RF million)	3,388.8	3,900.4	5,272.3	5,653.0	6,392.4	7,013.5	6,594.7	8,194.8	8,677.6
Salaries (RF million)	2,065.3	2,200.0	3,858.6	3,164.0	5,017.2	4,548.0	4,925.5	5,029.0	3,484.1
Allowances (RF million)	1009.0	1,361.0	1,171.3	2,212.0	1,132.1	2,216.0	1,383.1	2,851.0	4,714.4
Social security contributions (RF million)	201.3	216.0	136.5	165.0	153.2	164.0	125.7	153.0	214.4
Health care contributions made by the government for its employees (RF million)									
Total MINISANTE wage bill, including wage transfers (RF million)	113.2	123.0	105.9	111.0	89.9	87.0	160.4	162.0	264.8
Salaries (MINISANTE) (RF million)	2,135.6	2,656.8	3,318.2	3,994.1	3,619.0	4,638.1	4,230.5	3,123.5	1,303.0
Allowances (MINISANTE) (RF million)	1,214.7	1,387.0	2,292.3	1,957.0	2,669.3	2,652.0	3,280.8	2,908.0	863.6
Social security contributions (MINISANTE) (RF million)	708.9	1,043.0	884.4	1,873.0	827.0	1,848.0	837.5	893.0	339.8
	161.4	171.0	97.0	111.0	91.1	105.0	49.3	112.0	62.6

Health care contributions made by the government for its employees (MINISANTE) (RF million)	50.6	56.0	44.4	53.0	31.5	33.0	62.9	100.0	37.0
Total public payments to education human resources (RF million)	20,983.3	20,473.5	23,189.7	21,894.5	24,038.6	24,588.7	29,464.4	29,573.3	31,690.2
Salaries (RF million)	16,372.0	15,875.5	15,782.2	15,066.0	16,163.0	16,610.0	20,738.3	21,474.0	24,026.3
Allowances (RF million)	3,352.7	3,275.9	5,941.8	5,544.8	6,429.1	6,645.8	6,189.5	5,403.0	4,583.8
Social security contributions (RF million)	590.9	692.0	646.2	544.3	832.5	715.7	1,180.4	1,225.9	1,339.7
Health care contributions made by the government for its employees (RF million)	667.7	630.1	819.5	739.3	614.0	617.2	1,356.2	1,470.4	1,740.4
Total MINEDUC wage bill, including wage transfers (RF million)	6,431.7	6,307.6	7,854.7	6,508.5	6,655.4	6,705.5	9,274.0	9,313.4	10,408.4
Salaries (MINEDUC) (RF million)	5,404.4	5,215.9	4,609.1	3,538.8	3,121.9	3,094.8	5,786.0	6,578.0	9,642.0
Allowances (MINEDUC) (RF million)	850.5	896.9	3,179.7	2,873.1	3,299.1	3,347.5	2,880.6	1,871.6	35.0
Social security contributions (MINEDUC) (RF million)	93.5	103.0	20.3	44.1	83.6	96.3	353.9	492.9	400.2
Health care contributions made by the government for its employees (MINEDUC) (RF million)	83.3	91.8	45.6	52.6	150.8	166.9	253.5	370.9	331.2

(continued)

Annex Table 4.A.2   Database Used for Calculations, 2003-07 (Continued)

	2003		2004		2005		2006		2007
	Actual	Budget	Actual	Budget	Actual	Budget	Actual	Budget	Budget
Total number of civil servants paid through MIFOTRA (million)	39,676	39,676	37,156	37,156	39,507	39,507	40,063	40,063	
Health civil servants paid through MIFOTRA (million)					2,458	2,458	3,986	3,986	
Education civil servants paid through MIFOTRA (million)	31,318	31,318	32,236	32,236	33,278	33,278	34,571	34,571	
Total salaries paid through MIFOTRA (RF)	23,043,798,550	23,043,798,550	19,426,515,137	19,426,515,137	21,040,491,571	21,040,491,571	29,796,839,519	29,796,839,519	
Health salaries paid through MIFOTRA (RF)					2,576,588,478	2,576,588,478	3,263,082,681	3,263,082,681	
Education salaries paid through MIFOTRA (RF)	15,230,013,265	15,230,013,265	15,951,073,972	15,951,073,972	17,219,437,862	17,219,437,862	20,016,766,787	20,016,766,787	
Salary per civil servant paid by MIFOTRA (RF)	580,799	580,799	522,837	522,837	532,576	532,576	743,750	743,750	
Salary per health civil servant paid by MIFOTRA (RF)					1,048,246	1,048,246	818,636	818,636	
Salary per education civil servant paid by MIFOTRA (RF)	486,302	486,302	494,822	494,822	517,442	517,442	579,005	579,005	

Note: Author's calculation based on Ministry of Finance data.

Annex Figure 4.A.1   PBF Administrative and Oversight Structures for District Hospitals and Health Centers

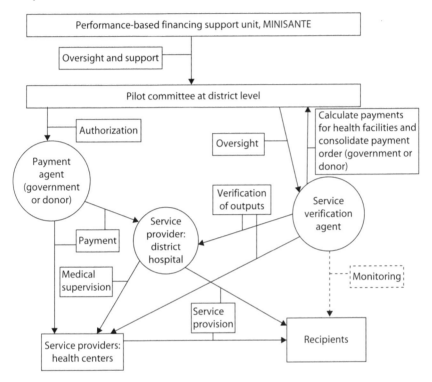

Source: MINISANTE 2006b.

Note: District hospital team is responsible for routine supervision of health centers for quality of care using standardized national supervisory checklists.

Annex Table 4.A.3   Annual Budget Preparation Schedule

Month	Stage	Districts	Line ministries	MINECOFIN	Development partners	Cabinet or Parliament
January	Joint review process (backward-looking review and orientations for next year)	**Annual district report** (explanation of budget execution relative to objectives)	Report on **annual execution plan and budget execution** (explanation of budget execution relative to objectives)	**Macroeconomic review and projections** (macroframework, estimation of overall resource envelope)		
February		**Joint district reviews**		**Annual economic report**	Participation in **joint district reviews**	**Akagera retreat**
March		Participation in **joint sector reviews**	**Joint sector reviews**	Consolidated **budget execution report**	Participation in **joint sector reviews**	
April			Participation in joint budget support and public financial management review	**Joint budget support and public financial management review**		
		.... Economic Development and Poverty Reduction Strategy annual progress report and summary of emerging priorities				
May	Strategic planning	Consultation with cells, sectors, and communities		**Budget call circular**	**Tentative statement of commitments**	
		Preparation of strategic issues papers[a]	**Preparation of strategic issues papers** (including provisional Medium-Term Expenditure Framework and earmarked transfers) (silent period for line ministries)			
June		**Meeting of network of planning and budgeting officers**		Preparation of first draft budget framework paper / Revision of macroframework and **budget revision**		
July		... **Budget consultations based on strategic issues papers and first draft budget framework paper** ... (Districts select representatives to attend sector consultations)	Sector consultations			

Budget preparation	August	Estimation of district revenues (taxes and donor funds)	Communication of final budget ceilings and earmarked grants		
			Data entry in Smartgov	**Finalization of budget framework** "Paper communication" of indicative transfers to districts	**Consultations with development partners, civil society, and the private sector**	**Cabinet discussion on budget framework paper**
		Preparation of **district budget framework paper**, including summary Medium-Term Expenditure Framework and key performance targets	Ministry Medium-Term Expenditure Framework finalized, including detailed budget			
	September	**Consultations, council scrutiny, and approval of summary Medium-Term Expenditure Framework**		Preparation of **draft Finance Law and explanatory note to the budget**	**Joint budget support and public financial management review** Agreement on Economic Development and Poverty Reduction Strategy Policy matrix	**Discussion of draft Finance Law by cabinet**
	October	**Preparation of detailed annual budget**			**Firm commitments for next year's budget**	**Discussion of draft Finance Law in Parliament**
	November					
	December	Council scrutiny and approval of **annual budget**				**Vote on Finance Law**

Source: Direction du Budget, MINECOFIN.

a. According to MINECOFIN (n.d.: 9), "The district projects revenues on the basis of grant ceilings provided by central government and its own estimates of local revenues and donor funding. Expenditure ceilings are provided to the different units, on the basis of which those units elaborate 3-year budget strategies, called Strategic Issues Papers (SIPs). This involves prioritisation of actions within the budget ceiling to make an optimal contribution to addressing local needs and national policy objectives. The Plan and Budget Working Group compiles the Local Government Budget Framework Paper (LGBFP), identifying key budgetary issues on the basis of unit SIPs."

Notes

1. This information was gathered during interviews with staff members of the Ministry of Public Service and Labour.

2. The index value refers to a harmonized multiplier that is applied to the salaries of health workers across the board, depending on where one works.

3. Because transfers to nonprofit private institutions appearing in the budgets include both salaries and functioning costs, they were not included in the calculations for this study; only subsidies to public institutions were included.

4. As shown later in the donor section, wages and salaries are also paid through the development budget, both by donors and by the government of Rwanda.

5. Under that subsection, four line items under the heading "Conditional support" are shown to health centers, health district centers, hospital districts, and reference hospitals, respectively.

6. Interview with the director of planning and policy, MINISANTE, February 2008.

7. Interestingly, the dip in 2005 coincides with the peak, in the same year, of the ratio of health expenditure over total government expenditure, reflecting the fact that the dip was attributable more to an increase in the denominator (total health expenditure), which occurred through a process independent of the wage bill process.

8. Interview with key staff members, MIFOTRA, February 2008.

9. Interview with the director of policy and planning, MINISANTE, February 2008.

10. This figure has been computed from table 6.3 of the EDPRS draft report.

11. For more information, see CEPEX's Web site at http://www.cepex.gov.rw/dgforeword.html.

12. An extrapolation of human resource expenditures, using the allocation to "salaries and allowances paid to human resources" of the amount pledged for 2006 as an indication of the relative size of salaries and allowances paid to the sector in the development budget, could give a rough estimate of the potential size of human resource expenditures in the development budgets. This amount might still be an underestimate, however, because some donors (such as the Global Fund to Fight AIDS, Tuberculosis, and Malaria) are known to have spent sizable amounts in human resource payments, even though actual figures are not known.

References

Fedelino, Annalisa, Gerd Schwartz, and Marijn Verhoeven. 2006. "Aid Scaling Up: Do Wage Bill Ceilings Stand in the Way?" IMF Working Paper 06/106, International Monetary Fund, Washington, DC. http://www.imf.org/external/pubs/ft/wp/2006/wp06106.pdf.

Furth, Rebecca, Robert Gass, and Jean Kagubare. 2005. "Rwanda Human Resources Assessment for HIV/AIDS Scale-UP. Phase 1 Report: National Human Resources Assessment." Prepared for the U.S. Agency for International Development by Quality Assurance Project, Bethesda, MD. http://www.qapro ject.org/pubs/PDFs/RwandaHRPhase1.pdf.

Goldsbrough, David, Tom Leeming, and Karen Christiansen. 2007. *IMF Programs and Health Spending: Case Study of Rwanda.* Washington, DC: Center for Global Development.

Herbst, Christopher. 2007. "Rwanda Health Worker Census." World Bank, Washington, DC.

IMF (International Monetary Fund). 2007a. "Rwanda: 2006 Article IV Consultation, First Review under the Three-Year Arrangement under the Poverty Reduction and Growth Facility, and Request for Waiver of Nonobservance of Performance Criteria—Staff Report; Staff Statement; Public Information Notice and Press Release on the Executive Board Discussion; and Statement by the Executive Director for Rwanda." IMF Country Report 07/80, IMF, Washington, DC.

———. 2007b. "Rwanda: Second Review under the Three-Year Arrangement under the Poverty Reduction and Growth Facility, Request for Waiver of Nonobservance of Performance Criterion, and Modification of Performance Criteria—Staff Report; Press Release on the Executive Board Discussion; and Statement by the Executive Director for Rwanda." IMF Country Report 07/233, IMF, Washington, DC.

MINECOFIN (Ministry of Finance and Economic Planning). 2007. *Economic Development and Poverty Reduction Strategy 2008–2012.* Kigali: MINECOFIN.

———. n.d. *Rwanda: Planning and Budgeting Guidelines for Local Governments, Volume 1: Guide to the District Community Development Planning and Budgeting Process.* Kigali: MINECOFIN.

MINEDUC (Ministry of Education). 2007. "Rwanda Public Expenditure Review, Education Sector." MINEDUC, Kigali.

MINISANTE (Ministry of Health). 2006a. *Human Resources for Health Strategic Plan 2006–2010.* Kigali: MINISANTE. http://www.moh.gov.rw/docs/Rwanda %20HRH%20strategic%20plan%20Final%20version-2010.pdf.

———. 2006b. "Performance Based Financing of Health Services in Rwanda: Development of a National PBF Model." Rwanda HIV Performance-Based Financing Project, Management Sciences for Health, Cambridge, MA. http://pdf.usaid.gov/pdf_docs/PNADI039.pdf.

———. 2007. "Solde Ligne de Dépenses 2007." MINISANTE, Kigale.

———. 2008. *Contractual Approach Guide for Health Centers: Utilization Manual.* Kigali: MINISANTE.

PEPFAR (President's Emergency Plan for AIDS Relief). 2007. *The Power of Partnerships: The President's Emergency Plan for AIDS Relief—Third Annual Report to Congress.* http://www.pepfar.gov/press/c19573.htm.

World Bank. 2007. *World Development Indicators 2007.* Washington, DC: World Bank.

CHAPTER 5

Background Country Study for the Dominican Republic

One of the key development priorities of the government of the Dominican Republic is to restructure its fiscal spending by cutting non-priority administrative expenditure and certain subsidies and using these savings to increase spending on health and education (Albizu, Montás, and Bengoa 2007: 4).

The health sector is going through a major reform process. Passed in 2001, the General Health Law and the Social Security Law mandate the transformation of the National Health System (NHS), including the organizational separation of financing from the service provision function. At the end of this process, the Ministry of Public Health and Social Assistance (Secretaría de Estado de Salud Pública y Asistencia Social, or SESPAS) will be left with the stewardship role for the sector, and the newly established National Insurance Agency will buy services from autonomous, regional health service networks.

The reform has major implications for the management of human resources for health (HRH). First, SESPAS has to develop a robust regulatory framework for HRH. Second, HRH management has to be transferred from SESPAS to regional health services. Third, regional health services have to build managerial HRH capacity to effectively respond to changes in demand for services.

In that connection, one key area of the government's strategy is to improve the performance of the health workforce. The Dominican Republic has a relatively large health workforce, with 3.8 health workers per 1,000 people. The primary issue is not an absolute shortage of health workers—although in some provinces, it is certainly a key issue—but the management of the health workforce and how performance can be improved. The efficiency with which the health sector allocates and implements its wage bill resources needs to be improved.

In the past five years, the Dominican Republic has gone through a series of macroeconomic reforms that have important implications for the health workforce. In 2002, the Dominican economy entered a recession. The country's public finances were placed under strain after the government bailed out the country's third-largest bank following a major fraud. This action consumed significant government resources and led to an economic crisis. By the end of 2003, inflation reached 42 percent, unemployment stood at 16.5 percent, and the Dominican peso (RD$) had lost more than half its value (Ribando 2005: 5).

As part of its fiscal response, the government implemented significant expenditure controls. One of the measures was a hiring freeze in the public sector. Interestingly, to partially reverse the recent compression in public sector real wages, the government increased nominal wages of central government employees by 30 percent. More important, the government's policy during this period of fiscal restraint was to protect spending in the social sectors—health and education (Albizu, Montás, and Bengoa 2005: 5).

The Health Wage Bill in the Dominican Republic

Most health workers are employed in the public sector in the Dominican Republic (in the NHS). Within the public sector, the largest employer is SESPAS, accounting for 64.6 percent of all health workers. The Social Security Institute (Istituto de Seguros Sociales, or IDSS) accounts for 25 percent, the private sector for 8.3 percent, the army for 0.8 percent, and nongovernmental organizations for 1.0 percent. The IDSS provider network will be integrated into the NHS umbrella. Currently, it is still separate because some issues remain to be resolved, such as the alignment of wage scales.

Each agency has different employment regulations and funding arrangements for health workers. This study limited its scope to the health workforce in SESPAS.

Process for Determining the Budget for the Health Wage Bill

Health workers employed in SESPAS are part of a national civil service. As a result, the health wage bill is paid from the public sector wage bill budget and is determined through a three-stage process.

When the government policy is to control spending on the public sector wage bill, the government will set a target level for the wage bill (covering all sectors), as it did after the financial crisis of 2002. In recent years, however, the size of the public sector wage bill has not posed any macroeconomic threat, and the government has not set any specific budget ceilings for the public sector wage bill (Albizu, Montás, and Bengoa 2007: 4). SESPAS is responsible for preparing the budget for the public sector based on the budgetary ceiling determined by the Ministry of Finance (MOF). Within this sector ceiling, SESPAS estimates the wage bill requirement for the sector, which is then included as a line item in the health budget. Sector budgets are consolidated, and negotiations within the government then determine the allocation of budgets to each sector, including the allocation of wage bill resources to particular sectors. Each of these stages is discussed. The process for determining the health wage bill is summarized in table 5.1.

Budget for the total public sector wage bill. Managing the size of the public sector wage bill level is important because it can cause macroeconomic volatility. High government wages and large employment can push up the wage bill and crowd out other spending. Government wage increases could feed into a general wage-price spiral that undermines competitiveness and could also result in fiscal slippages (Fedelino, Schwartz, and Verhoeven 2006).

Expansion of the public sector wage bill can limit fiscal space for implementing poverty reduction programs. However, it is equally important to strike a balance between macroeconomic targets and the need to increase budgets—including the wage bill—to expand coverage of key services to ensure the Dominican Republic achieves its development goals.

The Dominican Republic has a relatively small public sector wage bill relative to other countries in the region. As a percentage of gross domestic product (GDP), the public sector wage bill is quite low at 4.0 percent (figure 5.1). Figure 5.2 illustrates that the Dominican Republic public sector wage bill was 28 percent of total government expenditure in 2004, about average compared with other countries in the region.

As part of measures taken to resolve the financial crisis in 2002, the government implemented significant expenditure controls, including a hiring

Table 5.1 Process for Determining the Health Wage Bill

Actor	Process
Planning Office at SESPAS, Regional Health Directorate, and Regional Health Services at the health establishments	At the end of the first semester of every year, SESPAS evaluates the budget execution and the accomplishment of targets. This analysis allows budget reprogramming for the last trimester and the identification of new targets for the following year.
Ministry of Planning and Development	The ministry evaluates the sector budget execution and the deviation from the budget to plan for new fiscal ceilings.
Ministry of Planning and Development and sectors	The ministry discusses with each sector its plans for coverage increases or improvement of services.
Health minister, Planning Office at SESPAS, and directors of the different programs	Financial and physical targets are discussed and negotiated inside SESPAS between the health minister, the Planning Office, and the directors of the different programs to meet national and international development goals.
Health minister and Planning Office	Budget premises are defined (such as wage increases, budget allocation to certain areas), and a preliminary proposal for fiscal ceilings is established for the discussion with the president.
Planning Office at SESPAS	This stage occurs only within SESPAS and entails the Regional Health System. The discussion and negotiation process inside SESPAS begins. Training activities for budget formulation are implemented, and instructives and forms are given out to the Regional Health System stakeholders to start the budget formulation process.
Health minister, president, and professional associations	The health minister and president then negotiate with the different professional associations and unions regarding wage increases, incentives and post openings, training activities, and medical residencies, among other issues.

Planning Office at SESPAS	The office collects from local authorities the needs for infrastructure, equipment, and human resources.
NHS Planning Office, local authorities, and Ministry of Planning and Development	The NHS Planning Office consolidates the demands into a preliminary proposal. With this proposal, the internal and external negotiation process with (a) local authorities and unions and (b) the Ministry of Planning and Development starts.
National Office of Planning and National Office of the Budget	The two offices consolidate the final proposal.
National Development Council	The council is informed of the proposal.
Congress	Congress receives the budget proposal and at the same time receives demands from organized social groups. It approves the budget for each sector.
SESPAS	After the budget is negotiated with Ministry of Planning and Development and approved by Congress, SESPAS informs the different areas, services, and programs about the approved budget.
SESPAS and international cooperation agencies	SESPAS shares the budget with the international cooperation agencies and discusses the fiscal and physical targets to complement the budget with other sources of funding.

Source: Interviews conducted during the study.

Figure 5.1   Public Sector Wage Bill as a Share of GDP, by Country, 2005

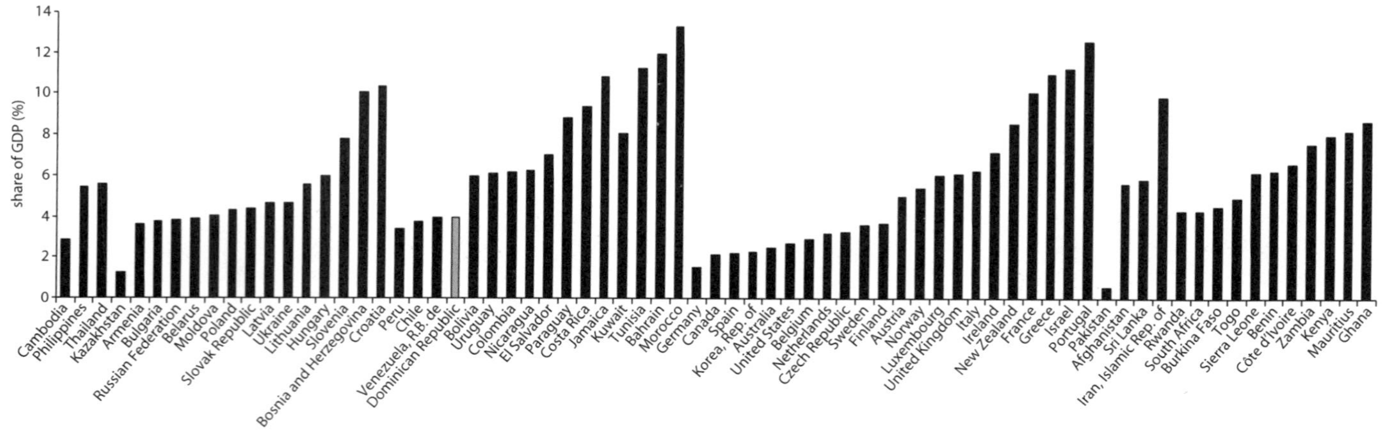

Share of GDP (%)

Countries (from top): Cambodia, Philippines, Thailand, Kazakhstan, Armenia, Bulgaria, Russian Federation, Belarus, Moldova, Poland, Slovak Republic, Latvia, Ukraine, Lithuania, Hungary, Slovenia, Bosnia and Herzegovina, Croatia, Peru, Chile, Venezuela, R. B. de, Dominican Republic, Bolivia, Uruguay, Colombia, Nicaragua, El Salvador, Paraguay, Costa Rica, Jamaica, Kuwait, Tunisia, Bahrain, Morocco, Germany, Canada, Spain, Korea, Rep. of, United States, Australia, Belgium, Netherlands, Czech Republic, Sweden, Finland, Austria, Norway, Luxembourg, United Kingdom, Italy, Ireland, New Zealand, France, Greece, Israel, Portugal, Pakistan, Afghanistan, Sri Lanka, Iran, Islamic Rep. of, Rwanda, South Africa, Burkina Faso, Sierra Leone, Togo, Benin, Côte d'Ivoire, Zambia, Kenya, Mauritius, Ghana

Source: World Bank 2007.

Figure 5.2   Public Sector Wage Bill as a Share of Government Expenditure, by Country, 2005

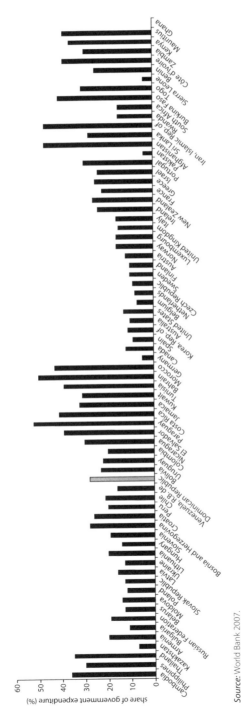

Source: World Bank 2007.

Note: These numbers are based on World Development Indicator data for total public sector compensation. The definition includes all payments in cash as well as in kind (such as food and housing) to employees in return for services rendered and government contributions to social insurance schemes such as social security and pensions that provide benefits to employees. Slight differences in the definition of total public sector compensation can account for the small variation from Dominican Republic data.

freeze in the public sector. The hiring freeze, which remained in effect until 2006, applied to all sectors; priority sectors had no exemptions (Albizu, Montás, and Bengoa 2006: 4).

In 2005, during the hiring freeze, the government increased nominal wages of government employees by 30 percent. In subsequent years, wages remained frozen for government employees but not for health workers and teachers. This policy was implemented to compensate for inflation and partially reverse compression in public sector wages that had occurred in the years leading up to the fiscal crisis. The wage increases applied to all sectors, and because inflation was 27 percent in 2003, 51 percent in 2004, and 4 percent in 2005, this increase in nominal wages was necessary and still did not keep pace with inflation.

In 2006, Congress approved the 2006 proposed budget, which specified a zero deficit in the public sector. The budget provided a series of measures, including (a) keeping nominal wages unchanged for most central government employees, except in the case of agreements reached with doctors and teachers; (b) containing administrative expenses; and (c) reducing subsidies. These measures were designed to offset increases in spending that were partly due to significant increases in social spending to achieve the Millennium Development Goals (Albizu, Montás, and Bengoa 2006: 2).

During the fiscal cutback period, the government aimed to prioritize spending in the health and education sectors. The government's policy during this period of fiscal restraint was to protect spending in health and education (Albizu, Montás, and Bengoa 2005: 5). As the analysis in later sections shows, this protection actually did happen with regard to the wage bill: the health and education sectors received an increasing portion of the overall wage bill.

Budget for the health sector wage bill. The budgeting of the health wage bill in SESPAS occurs in multiple stages. SESPAS receives a fiscal ceiling, including a wage bill line item. The wage bill ceiling is set in accordance with the expenditures in the previous year and estimates of government revenue. The resulting percentage increase varies from year to year, but it has been averaging about 3 percent. The ceiling may be altered during the budgeting process as a result of negotiations with unions. Within the fiscal ceilings set by the MOF, SESPAS prepares a budget that includes the wage bill as a line item.

Congress makes the final budgetary allocations to different ministries, including wage bill allocations. The negotiation stage takes place in

Congress, which has the ultimate decision-making authority on the government budget. In practice, Congress often adjusts fiscal ceilings during the negotiation stage. Congressional approval of the budget prepared by the MOF is not a mere formality.

Currently, no specific guidelines exist on how the wage bill budget in each sector should be determined, reflecting the fact that the public sector wage bill is not a major issue or concern to the government. In practice, SESPAS budgets for a small increase in the wage bill from year to year to cover annual wage increases for the current staffing contingent, historically about 3 percent per year. In the Dominican Republic, the number of unfilled vacancies is small, and staffing levels are deemed quite adequate. Thus, the only additional resources requested for the wage bill are to cover the annual wage increases and posts in newly established infrastructure.

According to policy, the health and education sectors have been singled out in recent years as priority sectors for additional wage bill resources. Earlier, no clear policy existed. In 2002 to 2005, during the overall hiring freeze, no explicit policy of exempting the health or education sector from the recruitment ban was in place, and the wage increase to the health and education sector was the same as for all civil servants. In 2006, however, doctors and teachers were exempted from the wage freeze that was implemented on all public sector employees.

The staffing levels in SESPAS are considered generally sufficient for delivering key services. It has no need for additional wage bill resources to increase staffing. Rather, wage bill resources are needed to pay higher salaries. Salaries for health workers are negotiated separately from those for administrative personnel, to whom a generic public sector wage scale applies. Pressures from labor conflicts are considered the most influential factor in determining salary levels and thus the budget and actual expenditures. Many unions and organized professional associations exist at the same time; the most important ones are the Dominican Medical Board (Colegio Médico Dominicano), the Health Unions Coordinator (Coordinadora de Gremios de la Salud), Odontologists Association (Asociación de Odontólogos), the Professional Nurses Association (Asociación de Enfermeras Graduadas), the Dominican Odontologist Association (Asociación Odontológica Dominicana), the Dominican Bioanalyst Association (Asociación Dominicana de Bioanalista), the Psychologists Association (Asociación Psicólogos), and the Dominican Pharmacist Association (Asociación Farmacéutica Dominicana).

Labor conflict is usually related to demands for job stability and better wage conditions that are not related to productivity or performance.

Authorities tend to accept these demands, given the social pressure and the potential for instability. Evidence shows an increase in expenses in the wage bill as a result of labor conflict and union agreements: in 2006, an increase of incentives for night shifts, distance, and years at work was successfully negotiated, and in 2007, a 20 percent increase in wages was agreed upon.

In sum, the public sector wage bill in health is primarily determined by (a) the historical budget for the wage bill, (b) additions to infrastructure, and (c) pressures from unions to increase salaries. Less important are international and national development targets.

Results of the Wage Bill Budgeting Process

The government of the Dominican Republic has decreased the share of its spending devoted to wages dramatically, dropping from 32.7 percent in 2002 to 20.8 percent in 2007 (figure 5.3). This decreasing trend shows that the government is not prioritizing the wage bill and instead is focusing its increased expenditure on nonwage areas. The government wage bill as a share of GDP demonstrates a similar trend. It declined from 6.8 percent in 2002 to 5.0 percent in 2006 (figure 5.4).

Figure 5.3   Public Sector Wage Bill as a Share of Government Expenditure, 2002–07

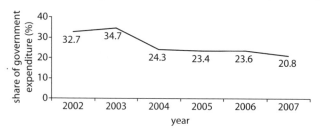

Source: Ministry of Finance.

Figure 5.4   Government Wage Bill as a Share of GDP, 2002–06

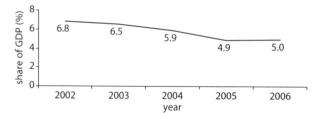

Source: Ministry of Finance.

Figure 5.5   Health Expenditure as a Share of Government Expenditure and Health Wage Bill as a Share of Health Expenditure, 2001–07

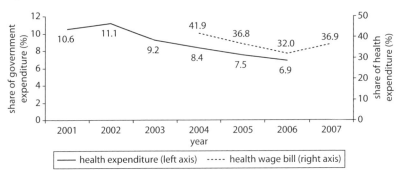

Sources: Budgets from the central government for 2002 to 2007, and from the National Office of the Budget and National Office of Planning of the Ministry of Economy, Planning and Development; from the Ministry of the Budget; and from the Central Bank of the Dominican Republic.

Government health expenditure as a share of government expenditure fell significantly during this same period, decreasing from 10.6 percent in 2001 to 6.9 percent in 2006 (see figure 5.5 and table 5.2). However, in real terms, government health spending increased from RD$6.8 million in 2001 to RD$16.4 million in 2006. The decline in health expenditure in relation to overall government expenditure shows that health was clearly not prioritized during this time and lost ground in relation to other sectors. Government health spending also fell in relation to GDP from 2001 to 2006, despite real GDP per capita increasing from RD$41,198 to RD$109,772.

In the Dominican Republic, 42 percent of the total budget in the health sector was allocated to salaries in 2004. This amount declined significantly to 32 percent in 2006.[1] The health sector wage bill is classically a big proportion of total health spending. Evidence shows that the wage bill in Latin American countries can reach 75 percent of the total budget in the health sector (Chen and others 2004). Although the wage bill constitutes a relatively large proportion of the SESPAS budget, the share of health spending going to wages has declined. This trend is projected to reverse between 2006 and 2007, with the health wage bill increasing to 37 percent of total health expenditure. The wage bill in the education sector also declined as a proportion of total government education spending, falling from 68.2 percent in 2004 to 59.1 percent in 2007 (figure 5.6). Education spending as a share of total government expenditure also fell from 2002 to 2005, showing that both the health

Table 5.2 Evolution of Public Spending in Health and Education, 2001–07

Type of expenditure	Amount (RD$ million), adjusted for inflation						
	2001	2002	2003	2004	2005	2006[a]	2007[a]
Total public expenditure	64,312.20	73,850.00	93,650.25	142,038.93	189,551.49	239,430.75	258,479.53
Total public health expenditure	6,786.60	7,777.20	6,332.40	9,632.50	13,886.00	16,411.70	19,557.90
Public health expenditure as a percentage of total public expenditure	10.55	10.53	6.76	6.78	7.33	6.85	7.57
Total public education expenditure	10,011.70	11,772.40	9,899.60	11,774.40	17,196.74	22,363.18	27,563.60
Public education expenditure as a percentage of total public expenditure	15.57	15.94	10.57	8.29	9.07	9.34	10.66
Real GDP	366,232.10	402,432.40	503,300.00	777,187.50	884,939.00	1,055,427.00	1,165,407.40
Public health expenditure as percentage of GDP	1.85	1.93	1.26	1.24	1.57	1.55	1.68

Sources: National Office of the Budget and National Office of Planning of the Ministry of Economy, Planning and Development; Ministry of the Budget; and Central Bank of the Dominican Republic.

a. Figures for these years are projections.

Figure 5.6   Education Expenditure as a Share of Government Expenditure and Education Wage Bill as a Share of Education Expenditure, 2001–07

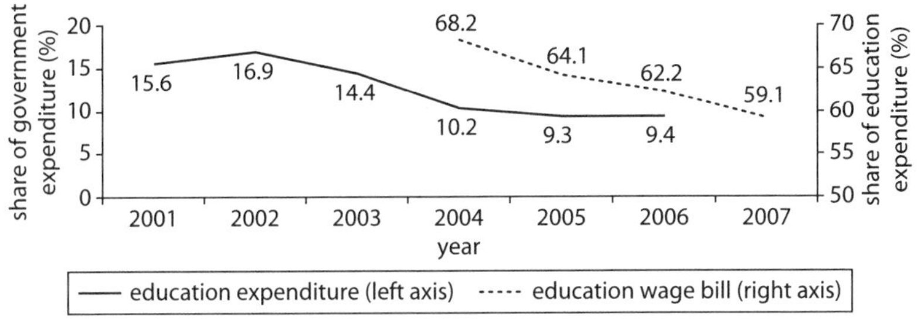

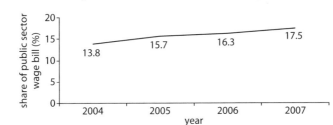

Sources: Budgets from the central government for 2002 to 2007, and from the National Office of the Budget and National Office of Planning of the Ministry of Economy, Planning and Development; from the Ministry of the Budget; and from the Central Bank of the Dominican Republic.

Figure 5.7   Health Wage Bill as a Share of Public Sector Wage Bill, 2004–07

Sources: Ministry of Finance and SESPAS.

and education sectors, which were supposed to be priority spending sectors for the government, were actually somewhat targeted.

The health wage bill has accounted for an increasing share of the public sector wage bill, which indicates that the health sector has been prioritized within the public sector wage bill. This share grew from 13.8 percent in 2004 to 17.5 percent in 2007 (figure 5.7). While the government was cutting the public sector wage bill, the health sector seems to have been insulated from these reductions. The education sector again mirrors the experience of the health sector. The education wage bill as a share of the public sector wage bill increased from 22.7 percent in 2004 to 27.8 percent in 2007 (figure 5.8). As expected, the education wage bill is a larger proportion of the public sector wage bill than health because education is a more labor-intensive sector. Thus, the public sector wage bill decline has been focused on sectors other than education

Figure 5.8   Education Wage Bill as a Share of Public Sector Wage Bill, 2004–07

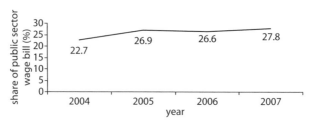

Sources: Ministry of Finance and SESPAS.

Figure 5.9   Distribution of Public Sector Wage Bill, by Sector, 2005 and 2007

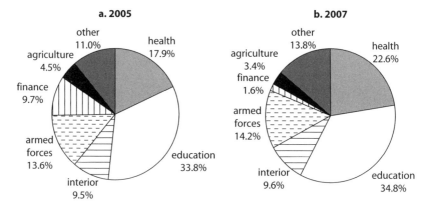

Source: Central Bank of the Dominican Republic.

and health. Although health spending has declined, the health sector has been prioritized within the overall civil service.

The main conclusion is that health has been prioritized in terms of the public sector wage bill. However, this prioritization was not sufficient to maintain a constant ratio of wage-to-nonwage spending within the health sector. Moreover, had health spending not fallen as dramatically as it did, the ratio of wage-to-nonwage spending would have declined even further. This finding suggests that public sector wage bill policy could be an important factor constraining expansion of the health wage bill. The prioritization of health and education in the wage bill came mainly at the expense of the MOF and the Ministry of Agriculture (figure 5.9).

Budget execution of salaries is very high in SESPAS; however, execution of other remuneration, particularly allowances and incentives, is extremely unreliable and scattered (table 5.3). Budget execution of the

Table 5.3 Budgeted and Executed Wage Bill at SESPAS, 2004–06

Wage bill structure	2004 wage bill			2005 wage bill			2006 wage bill		
	Budgeted (RD$)	Executed (RD$)	Percentage of budget	Budgeted (RD$)	Executed (RD$)	Percentage of budget	Budgeted (RD$)	Executed (RD$)	Percentage of budget
Total									
remuneration	4,103,800,868	3,918,506,896	95	5,938,899,713	5,618,627,719	95	7,205,007,654	6,127,828,667	85
Permanent staff	3,102,589,884	2,876,674,890	93	4,213,503,467	4,307,617,088	102	5,230,025,795	3,773,467,514	72
Short-term personnel	208,644,059	222,381,507	107	465,178,272	361,586,163	78	601,575,339	508,098,284	84
Allowances and incentives	74,417,228	216,969,683	292	330,299,316	350,527,731	106	883,613,524	862,440,058	98
Seniority	0	211,559,821		0	39,320		0	33,832	
Compensation for food expenses	0	0	0	0	0		0	231,044	
Compensation for extra hours	0	2,294,015					0	495,917,976	
Compensation for other services	0	3,115,847			6,035,942		0	0	
Contractor fees	179,145,535	22,330,648	12	169,254,534	69,022,291	41	139,024,869	77,947,344	56
Representation expenses	0	1,149,973		1,379,968	1,365,926	99	1,925,711	0	0

(continued)

179

Table 5.3 Budgeted and Executed Wage Bill at SESPAS, 2004–06(Continued)

Wage bill structure	2004 wage bill			2005 wage bill			2006 wage bill		
	Budgeted (RD$)	Executed (RD$)	Percentage of budget	Budgeted (RD$)	Executed (RD$)	Percentage of budget	Budgeted (RD$)	Executed (RD$)	Percentage of budget
Benefits	257,254,106	259,036,896	101	223,513,095	283,562,164	127	0	525,880,413	
Social security contributions	281,750,056	102,993,616	37	535,771,061	238,871,094	45	348,842,416	379,995,054	109
Allowances and Incentives	74,417,228	216,969,683	292	330,299,316	350,527,731	106	883,613,524	862,440,058	98
Seniority		211,559,821		0	39,320		0	33,832	
Compensation for food expenses		0		0	0		0	231,044	
Compensation for extra hours		2,294,015		0			0	495,917,976	

Sources: National Office of the Budget, Ministry of the Budget, and SESPAS.

salaries for all types of workers remains very close to 100 percent from 2004 through 2006. However, budget execution of allowances and incentives ranges from 292 percent to 85 percent. The wage bill structure comprises wages for workers with tenure, wages for workers with short-term contracts, allowances and incentives, seniority in the job, extra hours at work, fees for services, representation expenses, benefits, and social security contributions. A large proportion of the health workforce wages corresponds to workers with permanent contracts. In 2006, about 76 percent of payroll spending went to workers with permanent contracts, while about 9 percent of the budget was allocated to pay workers with more flexible contractual mechanisms, and another 2 percent of the wage bill went to pay for allowances, which include recognition of extra hours and years at work.

The overruns in budget execution for allowances and incentives are not surprising, given the leeway SESPAS has to negotiate these amounts throughout the year with labor unions. SESPAS is able to reallocate funds from other areas of its budget to pay for additional allowances and incentives not previously in the budget. As seen in table 5.3, the amount budgeted for allowances and incentives increased dramatically from 2004 to 2006 as a result of negotiations with labor unions and large budget overruns in 2004.

Since 2005, recruitment of staff has fallen within SESPAS (table 5.4). In 2005, 2,278 staff members were recruited into SESPAS, falling to 1,860 in 2007 and 1,857 in 2008. These recruitment levels resulted in a net increase of staff of 2,073 in 2005, falling to just over 1,000 in 2008. Clearly, net recruitment levels are falling significantly within SESPAS, but as indicated earlier, the government's HRH strategy is not focused on scaling up the health workforce.

Table 5.4   Recruitment and Separation of Staff in SESPAS, 2005–08

	2005	2006	2007	2008
Total recruitment of personnel	2,278	2,704	1,860	1,857
Total separations of personnel	205	1,554	1,829	835
Net recruitment of personnel	2,073	1,150	31	1,022

Source: SESPAS.

Public Sector Employment of Health Workers

Within a given wage bill envelope, identifying areas where SESPAS can improve the efficiency of how wage bill resources are spent is important. The budget for the health wage bill comes out of the budget for the public sector wage bill. Thus, the health wage bill will always be constrained by the size of the public sector wage bill. In the future, the health sector needs to make the best use of existing resources. There is increasing consensus that restrictive contracting arrangements, rigidity in labor mobility, and a fixed structure of wages without incentive mechanisms are potential barriers to improving health workforce performance.

In the context of the Dominican Republic, 13 different procedures related to contracting arrangements, labor mobility, and allowances have been identified, among them, the Regulation for Human Resources for Health in the National Health System and the General Hospital Regulation. These regulations contain policies that regulate the hiring process of HRH, mobility, wages and post classification system, selection and recruitment, incentives and allowances, performance evaluation, and promotion.

This section describes how health workers are currently recruited, deployed, and managed in the public sector.

Creating Funded Posts in the Health Sector

SESPAS and other public institutions in the health sector define the number of posts for each professional category on the basis of a Post Map of health centers. This information is derived from input given by the directors of each health center, who are supposed to base their estimates on overall demand and needs. However, requests for additional posts from the local health centers are commonly ignored. Therefore, most additional posts are created at the central level and do not necessarily reflect the needs of the health centers.

In practice, most health posts are created as a result of either the construction of a new health facility or the departure of a current health worker. No large scaling-up effort is evident in the number of health workers. The public recruitment process is not based on an evaluation of needs and demands, and it is not strategically planned. This situation may change soon, however. The General Health Law and the Social Security Law place particular emphasis on primary health care. Most important, primary health care facilities will have gatekeeper functions. Therefore, a major effort can be anticipated to strengthen primary care services, including their staff base.

Before being approved by the MOF and subsequently filled, new positions as well as vacancies have to be confirmed by the Office of Personnel Management. Although this procedure provides a mechanism to control the wage bill and, furthermore, to ensure the efficient allocation of resources, confirmation criteria for the approval of new positions and vacancies have yet to be established and enforced.

Currently, the Office of Personnel Management is working to address these deficiencies by developing four distinct human resources policies for education, judiciary, health, and foreign affairs that will be independent from the law for civil servants. The intent of these policies is not only to make human resource management procedures more effective and transparent but also to define wage scales and career paths and to strengthen workforce planning.

Recruiting Health Workers in the Public Sector

Recruitment of health workers into funded posts is supposed to be managed regionally; however, in practice, most of the selection and recruitment processes are carried out at the central level. In only very few cases, the recruitment process follows a public selection process prescribed by the overall civil service recruitment procedures. Job openings are not typically advertised. Although SESPAS makes the final decision on selecting and appointing staff members, regions very often provide a short list of candidates and a recommendation for the top choice. The State Department approves SESPAS's selection, although this step is a formality. No data are available on the time that filling a position takes.

The recruitment process is heavily influenced by pressures from various professional associations and unions. The process is supposed to be based on objective criteria, including experience, background, continuing education and training, and research activities. Nevertheless, no public recruitments have been held in seven years to hire specialists (OPS 2007: 27) in the health sector. Only in a few cases was the selection process based on approved terms of reference and an evaluation process.

The Office of Human Resources for Health in SESPAS, which is supposed to regulate the hiring mechanisms for the health workforce, is currently concentrated on regulating the movements within SESPAS itself. In practice, the hiring process depends on the amount of the budget rather than planned increases in funded posts. This system provides a high level of discretion both in the selection process and in negotiations of the individual's salary and benefits.

Table 5.5   Skill Mix of Human Resources for Health, 2004–06

Health worker category	2004	2005	2006
Doctors	9,204	10,572	10,380
Nurses	11,333	11,093	12,088
Specialists	1,414	1,164	1,166
Psychologists	250	133	288
Pharmacists	527	588	619
Radiologists	61	163	200
Dentists and dental assistants	1,431	1,430	1,276
Other health personnel	5,875	3,172	4,091
Total health personnel	30,095	28,315	30,108

Source: SESPAS.

Because of weak strategic planning, the skill mix and geographic distribution of health workers is very poor (table 5.5). The proportion of untrained personnel among doctors and nurses is high. In 2005, according to SESPAS, 80 percent of nurses were assistant nurses and 25 percent of physicians were interns or residents. Additionally, relatively few licensed nurses exist when compared with physicians. The ratio of doctors (excluding interns and residents) to licensed nurses was 3.6:1 in 2006. The increasing number of assistant nurses, who are less expensive, suggests that less trained personnel could be replacing licensed nurses.

Human resources for health are concentrated in a few provinces in the Dominican Republic. This inequitable distribution is seen in table 5.6. Large variations in staffing levels are observed, especially among doctors and assistants.

The available information on skill mix, deployment, and distribution of health workers is incomplete and scattered. Even though SESPAS has a planning tool for human resources and equipment related to health needs, this tool has not been updated over the years. Hence, the information system currently in use is highly deficient and unsuitable for planning and management of HRH. Given this situation, the planning process for health workers in SESPAS is certainly not related to the identification of health demands or planning for adequate deployment and distribution of health workers around the country.

Even though some managerial instruments were identified, little coordination exists between these instruments, and they are out of date. Instruments include strategic planning for HRH and for the development of service networks as well as the identification of gaps between staffing and needs. Moreover, the planning process is subject to strong pressures from unions and politics. The actual recruitment process and the way in

Table 5.6   Concentration of Health Workers in Provinces, 2003

				Number of health workers per 10,000 inhabitants					
Province	Doctors	Professional Nurses	Pharmacists	Assistants	Bioanalysts	Odontologists	Psychologists	Other	Veterinarians
Azua	146	7	3	279	16	10	1	4	0
Bahoruco	67	16	3	217	23	8	2	2	0
Barahona	151	38	3	422	25	12	1	6	2
Dajabón	56	10	3	178	5	10	0	3	0
Distrito Nacional	3,886	602	82	3,823	540	612	178	39	16
Duarte	296	85	4	563	30	24	5	2	1
El Seibo	86	11	2	123	5	6	0	3	0
Elías Piña	44	4	3	156	6	4	0	6	1
Espaillat	144	27	4	267	9	14	2	11	0
Hato Mayor	102	5	1	125	9	9	1	0	0
Independencia	51	8	2	208	9	3	1	3	1
La Altagracia	126	12	2	107	15	18	1	3	0
La Romana	127	12	1	122	9	15	1	1	0
La Vega	300	32	5	484	40	46	7	5	2
María Trinidad Sánchez	116	14	8	263	9	17	0	1	0
Monseñor Nouel	145	13	2	185	15	13	3	1	0
Monte Cristi	103	7	9	240	10	13	1	3	0
Monte Plata	132	5	5	171	7	14	2	1	0
Pedernales	23	2	1	40	2	2	0	1	0
Peravia	172	27	3	248	10	12	0	2	0
Puerto Plata	200	24	5	330	16	27	3	7	0
Salcedo	110	27	3	354	21	18	6	1	1

(continued)

Table 5.6 Concentration of Health Workers in Provinces, 2003(Continued)

Province		Doctors	Professional Nurses	Pharmacists	Assistants	Bioanalysts	Odontologists	Psychologists	Other	Veterinarians
					Number of health workers per 10,000 inhabitants					
Samaná		84	8	4	181	21	7	1	1	0
San Cristóbal		395	89	8	533	38	33	5	5	0
San José de Ocoa		71	5	2	122	5	6	0	0	0
San Juan		195	35	2	555	13	26	2	8	1
San Pedro de Macorís		395	46	11	315	32	39	1	8	1
Sánchez Ramírez		137	22	3	277	19	13	0	1	1
Santiago		949	106	17	1,114	112	93	19	9	4
Santiago Rodríguez		60	13	2	166	8	7	0	4	0
Santo Domingo		0	0	0	0	0	0	0	0	0
Valverde		109	27	2	180	7	13	3	0	1
Country		8,978	1,339	205	12,348	1,086	1,144	246	141	32
Total		35.2%	5.2%	0.8%	48.4%	4.3%	4.5%	1.0%	0.6%	0.1%

Source: Executive Commission for Reform of the Health Sector.

Note: Examples of rural and underdeveloped provinces with household incomes below the national average include Dajabón, Barahona, Bahoruco, Monte Plata, La Altagracia, and Elías Piña.

Table 5.7   Main Actors and Their Roles in the Process for Labor Mobility

Main actor	Process
Health worker	Makes requests to his or her superior to transfer to another health center. This request is then sent to the health center in question.
Health center director	Sends the request to the minister of health through the Office of Human Resources for Health in SESPAS, recommending worker be hired.
Office of Human Resources for Health in SESPAS	Verifies the vacancy of a funded post and evaluates the need to fill the post. If the need is approved, the office sends the request to the minister of health.
Minister of Health	Approves the request and informs the Office of Human Resources for Health.

Source: Interviews conducted during the study.

which the selection process is managed leads to large inefficiencies in the public sector health workforce.

Many actors and steps are involved for a health worker to transfer to another health center, thus creating distortions in the transfer system. Table 5.7 describes the various actors involved in the process. In theory, to transfer to another post, a health worker has to enter into an entirely new recruitment process and therefore find a new or vacated post to apply to. Furthermore, movements from outside the capital to Santo Domingo are strictly forbidden, given the shortages of HRH around the country. However, if they are already based in Santo Domingo, staff members are allowed to transfer outside the capital city. In practice, labor mobility is not necessarily related to distribution or needs, and transfers are usually allowed for reasons other than health priorities. To assist in assessing staffing needs, SESPAS has initiated a mapping study, which will be completed before the end of the year.

Terms of Work in the Public Sector

Terms of work include tenure, remuneration, promotion, and termination and sanctions.

Tenure. Within SESPAS, two main types of contracts are specified in the legal framework (that is, article 19 of the Regulation for Human Resources for Health in the National Health System):

- Short-term contracts, which are annual contracts that can be renewed
- Ordinary contracts, which in practice are permanent and pensionable, although the contract does not specify the length of service

The majority of employees in SESPAS are on permanent and pensionable contracts. A large proportion of the health workforce's wages corresponds to workers with permanent contracts. In 2006, about 76 percent of the health wage bill was accounted for by health workers with permanent contracts. Short-term contract employees accounted for only about 9 percent of the health wage bill.

Short-term contracts are used to a much larger extent than policy allows. According to SEPSAS regulations, short-term contracts should be exclusively used in cases where posts are vacant for specific reasons, such as temporary leave for medical reasons, for maternity, or because of transfer to an administrative position. Ordinary contracts guarantee job stability and therefore the right to pensions, allowances, and other benefits. In practice, short-term contracts are used widely. For example, they are used to employ medical residents who are not covered by SESPAS employment regulations. They are also used to cope with inflexible hiring mechanisms and to pay for extra time. In contrast to ordinary contracts, for example, the number of hours worked under short-term contracts is not regulated, and flexible terms are used.

The employment of medical residents and medical students is not regulated, but in practice they are an important source of HRH and are usually employed on short-term contracts. In recent years, a sustained effort has been made to use medical residents or medical students instead of doctors to deliver services at the primary care level, particularly in underserviced areas, often because doctors are not willing to work in these areas even though positions are funded. Besides not having the proper medical background to guarantee adequate provision of health services, medical residents or students may constitute a limitation in terms of service, because they are not allowed to prescribe medicines or diagnostic tests. The government is currently establishing estimates of the staffing gap in underserviced areas and has commissioned work to render the current incentive scheme for rural areas more effective.

The required hours of work specified in the labor regulations is quite low and falling. Under ordinary contracts, health workers used to be required to work a minimum of 6 hours per day and a maximum of 30 hours per week. In response to the last health workers' strike, new contractual agreements have reduced these limits to a maximum of 20 hours of work per week—effectively a 33 percent increase in hourly wages. The labor unions and SESPAS are finding creative ways to increase remuneration. In situations where SESPAS is able to secure additional wage bill resources for the health sector, the union pressures for increased wages are met with an increase in salary levels. In situations where SESPAS cannot secure additional wage bill resources, the union demands are met through reductions in hours worked. Both policy responses increase the hourly wage of health workers, but they have very different implications for the actual labor supply available in public facilities.

With reductions in maximum hours worked, health workers spend less time working in SESPAS facilities and more time working in the private sector. Dual practice is common in the Dominican health sector and in the Latin American and Caribbean region in general (Ferrinho and others 2004). With reductions in maximum hours worked, health care workers are able to increase their take-home pay by simply devoting more hours to dual practice. With the rollout of the National Insurance Scheme (NIS), the reduction in maximum hours worked is even more important to health workers, especially doctors. The NIS is expected to increase the demand for health services—and thus, for doctors—among the poor, who are currently being enrolled in the subsidized regime of National Family Insurance. Because the insurance scheme pays doctors on a fee-for-service basis, income opportunities associated with working in the private sector are considerable.

The focus of union demands has shifted with the plan to implement the NIS. Union pressures were focused on increasing salary levels. When persistent salary increases became unaffordable and SESPAS resisted, unions demanded reductions in hours worked. Now, with the maximum hours worked per week down to 20 hours, unions are focusing on lobbying to increase the fee schedule within the NIS. Given the increased hours available for dual practice in the private sector, increasing the fees will have a very large effect on income. Although this development will likely relieve some of the pressure on SESPAS to pay higher salaries, it will generate cost escalation within the NIS.

Remuneration. Health workers receive three types of remuneration: salaries, allowances, and incentives. According to SESPAS policy, salaries are determined by job characteristics; however, this policy is not strictly followed. Salaries vary widely from region to region, from individual to individual, and among individuals with the same responsibilities. The salary scale is not framed within the post classification system, meaning that no formal relation exists between salaries and job characteristics. Likewise, allowances and incentives are not paid according to SESPAS policies. A recent evaluation of the distribution of earnings within SESPAS shows a variety of inconsistencies in salaries, allowances, and incentives.

Table 5.8   Average Monthly Salaries for Health Workers in SESPAS, 2001–05

Health worker category	Amount (RD$, adjusted for inflation)				
	2001	2002	2003	2004	2005
General physicians	11,950	11,965	9,269	11,195	17,439
Specialists	12,804	12,819	9,931	11,995	18,660
Medical residents	8,251	8,261	6,400	7,092	11,047
Graduate interns	11,381	11,395	8,827	9,782	15,237
Licensed nurses	5,928	5,935	4,598	5,553	8,650
Assistant nurses	4,869	4,879	3,780	4,565	7,111
Bioanalysts	5,691	5,697	4,414	5,331	8,304
Psychologists	5,928	5,935	4,598	5,553	8,650
Pharmacists	5,928	5,935	4,598	5,553	8,650
Social workers	2,034	2,036	1,577	1,905	2,968

Source: SESPAS.

There are considerable differences in salaries for the same position, even within the same facility, in contradiction to the regulation. Variations in earnings are even more pronounced; for example, in the same health center, unlicensed nurses have earnings from RD$2,039 to RD$17,793.[2]

Unions play a major role in setting salary levels in the health sector. The salary scale for the health sector is separate from that of the civil service in general. Thus, SESPAS is free to change salary levels without any spillover effects into other sectors. Unions are very powerful in salary negotiations. Each year, within the budget cycle, the labor unions for each professional category negotiate with SESPAS to determine the salary levels of health workers. Strikes are very common in the Dominican Republic, as in the region in general, and the threat of strikes is a powerful force in shaping salary levels of health workers (Novick and Rosales 2006).

Real salary levels have increased in recent years, roughly at the same rate for all categories of health workers. Among the different health categories, physicians have the highest salary, followed by medical residents and graduate interns. Doctors make about twice the salary of nurses (see table 5.8). Real wages increased between 2001 and 2005 by 45 percent for both nurses and doctors.

The increasing trend in health workers' salaries is consistent with increases in other sectors' wages. As shown in figure 5.10, health and education salaries are relatively comparable to wages in public administration, utilities and transport, and skilled services. These trends show that the increases in health wages between 2000 and 2006 are not specific to the health sector and instead reflect public sector wage bill pressures throughout the Dominican Republic.

Figure 5.10   Hourly Wage Comparison, 2000–06

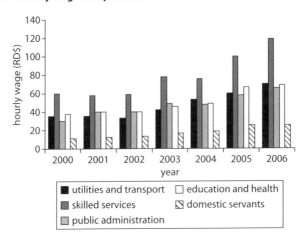

Source: Socio-Economic Database for Latin America and the Caribbean, http://www.depeco.econo.unlp.edu.ar/cedlas/sedlac/.

Allowances make up a significant share of the overall earnings for health workers in SESPAS. In 2006, allowances and incentives constituted 14 percent of the overall wage bill. According to Article 20 of the Regulation for Human Resources for Health in the National Health System, health workers are entitled to certain allowances in addition to their regular salary. The purpose of these allowances is to attract, retain, motivate, and compensate health workers and to reward those who are outstanding and highly motivated. There are four primary categories of allowances. Fixed allowances are applied on the basis of seniority in the job and according to geographic location of the position. Variable allowances are based on performance and extra hours worked; they can vary across districts as well as from year to year. Short-term staff members do not receive allowances or incentives.

Fixed allowances are used to compensate those employees who work in more remote areas as well as to reward employees for years of service worked; they are included in the Regulation for Human Resources for Health in the National Health System. Allowances for years worked are relatively small and grow at a slow rate. As seen in figure 5.11, the seniority allowance does not begin until after 14 years of service for assistant doctors. Once a doctor puts in 14 years of service, he or she receives additional allowances for every 5 years of service after that point. Health workers have to work for many years to be so rewarded. For nurses, initial

Figure 5.11   Salaries and Incentives for Years at Work for Assistant Doctors

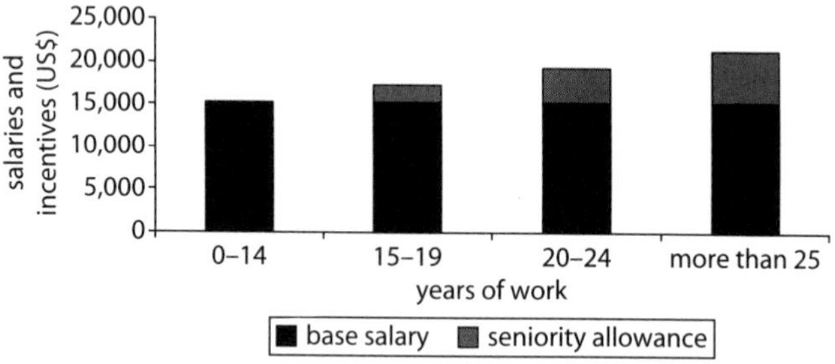

Source: SESPAS, May 2007.

allowances are given after 5 years of service, but they do not increase again until a nurse reaches 20 years of service. For assistant doctors and nurses working more than 25 years, the seniority allowance is 28 percent of their total compensation.

As in the case of salaries, allowances are subject to negotiations with unions. Results of negotiations are recorded in agreements signed by the unions and the government. Agreements vary from union to union; thus, allowances vary from cadre to cadre.

According to policy, allowances for working in certain geographic locations are supposed to be tied to the location, but in practice they are not. In contrast with the allowance for years of work, the geographic allowance is tied to certain positions in geographic areas. Rural allowances vary from cadre to cadre, as well as across locations. The allowance applies both to a newly hired staff member who fills a vacant position in a certain area and to a health worker who is transferred to a location eligible for the allowance. In practice, when the person leaves the location, the allowance turns into a permanent component of the worker's wage. This practice generates distortions in the objectives of the allowance. It also generates significant upward pressure on the budget allocated for rural allowances, because people keep claiming them even after leaving the original position. Additionally, the rural allowance is not enough to motivate health workers to reside and practice away from Santo Domingo.

Rural hardship allowances are provided to attract staff members to hardship areas, but these allowances are small relative to overall compensation. According to key informants, the allowances are unlikely to be adequate as a financial incentive for attracting staff members to these areas.

Variable allowances include incentives for good performance and working extra hours. These allowances are unpredictable and can vary greatly both across districts and from year to year. Furthermore, in many instances they come as a result of union pressure and the threat of strikes by doctors. No clear regulation exists governing the amount of either of these two allowances, thus giving discretion to SESPAS to adjust them in accordance with the level of union pressure applied on an annual basis. The threat of strike by doctors is a predictable, annual event. Therefore, SESPAS expects that it will be forced to negotiate the level of these allowances on the basis of the pressure applied. This money is not allocated specifically for allowances in the budget; therefore, SESPAS funds it by reallocating funds away from other activities through a series of special transfers.

SESPAS has worked to develop a comprehensive framework for the performance-based allowance; however, it has never been fully implemented. Currently, much of the performance-based incentive scheme centers around institutional goals that are set with SESPAS. On the basis of a number of benchmarks, including number of patients seen, types of services provided, and level of facility, health facilities receive a certain amount of additional funds. These incentives are given as a fixed amount per person and as a percentage of the cost of a particular service, and they vary by type of facility. For instance, a specialized health center receives 7 percent of services provided, whereas a basic health center receives 5 percent of services provided. The scheme has never been implemented, and SESPAS is currently revising it.

The distribution and level of the allowance for extra hours worked allow the most discretion. For instance, evidence shows a dramatic increase of allowances in the form of recognized extra hours. These have increased from 2 percent of the total remuneration budget in 2004 to 14 percent in 2006. This large variation indicates this is the allowance the unions have the greatest power to influence through strike threats and other pressure. Given that health workers are required to work only 20 hours per week, unions can lobby to receive extra pay for a lot of potential extra hours.

Allowances do not provide clear incentives to health workers. In addition to the poor incentive structure, the implementation of the allowance scheme lacks transparency and equality. The seniority allowance is given only to those workers who have been working for 14 years or more, thus assuming that health workers will approach their careers on a long-term horizon. The rural allowance is not enough to draw workers outside Santo Domingo. The variable allowances are used as a way to appease union pressures instead of as a reward for performance or for working extra hours.

Promotion. The Regulation for Human Resources for Health in the National Health System states that promotions are to be governed by a performance evaluation system; however, because a performance evaluation system has never been fully implemented, promotions are based on other factors. Furthermore, the regulation lists a total of nine different steps of approval for a promotion to be granted. This intense level of bureaucracy makes receiving a timely promotion seem very difficult. Although SESPAS recognizes the need to change to a performance evaluation system, the lack of implementation can lead to low morale and frustration among health workers. Key informants suggested that promotion is based mainly on seniority and political favoritism. In addition, higher-level promotions are made directly by the president and are often independent of performance. The result is that high-level staff members have very short tenure, changing every four years or so.

Termination and sanctioning. A termination and sanctioning policy currently exists, but it is not followed. The employment regulations define conditions for contract termination. They clearly state that it will happen only in the event of disciplinary sanction, retirement, or voluntary termination of the contract. In practice, however, there is no evidence of significant layoffs among health workers as a result of sanctioning.

Key Messages

In response to an economic crisis and in line with recommendations of the International Monetary Fund (IMF), the government significantly reduced the size of the public sector wage bill. These wage bill cuts affected the health sector, but not as severely as other sectors.

The health sector accounted for a steadily increasing share of the overall wage bill. During the economic crisis, IMF recommendations were limited to targets for the public sector wage bill. In line with the wage bill targets, the government set sector-specific targets. No clear policy indicated which sectors were to be prioritized both during and after the economic crisis.

The health wage bill budgetory process is not very strategic and is politically driven. The experience highlights the importance of the budgeting process for allocating wage bill resources to different sectors. The health sector can be more strategic in its negotiations. It has to be seen how the new budget law will affect this process. In general, the new law stipulates the preparation of a results-based national development plan that will serve as the strategic framework for the annual budgeting process.

Not only for health but for all sectors, the budgeting process implies setting separate thresholds for the wage bill and nonwage expenditure, leaving SESPAS and regional health services with no control over how to allocate health spending resources across labor and nonlabor inputs. As a result, the share of nonwage health spending has fallen, despite more public sector wage bill resources being devoted to the wage bill. Whether this trend has had any significant implications for service delivery is unclear.

The final budget decision rests with Congress. In this approval process, strategic budget plans run the risk of being distorted by priorities set by parties and by pressures from local constituencies and labor unions.

In the absence of an explicit HRH strategy, wage bill resources have been used primarily to ensure that facilities are appropriately staffed. Unlike many other developing countries, the Dominican Republic has achieved almost universal geographic access to health services. Therefore, the government has made no major push to scale up staffing levels.

The Dominican Republic has one of the highest physicians per nurse ratios in the world. Partially the result of policies influenced by labor unions, this skill mix results in inefficiencies and is not conducive to the government's goal of strengthening primary care.

The government has had no explicit, comprehensive government strategy for HRH. In the absence of such a strategy, wage bill resources have been primarily used to ensure a minimum staffing of the public network of health facilities.

Negotiations between the government and labor unions have shifted to focusing on hours worked. Having approved a 10-year plan for the health sector, the government aims to develop an HRH strategy shortly. The development of such a strategy will, however, be hampered by a dearth of information on the performance of the workforce, including data on its size and distribution.

Limits on the expansion of the health wage bill, upward pressures on salaries from labor unions, and the implicit government strategy to ensure minimum staffing levels of the public health service network have led to several important developments in the labor market. Even though health has been prioritized within the overall wage bill, the health wage bill has not been growing fast enough to meet the salary demands of labor unions. The maximum hours worked stipulated in public sector contracts for health workers has decreased significantly to 20 hours per week. With such a low level reached, future upward salary pressures are unlikely to be diffused through decreases in hours worked.

Reduction of hours worked, in turn, has only been possible because the private sector is well developed and dual practice is prominent. With private sector work opportunities mainly located in urban areas, the current low-level equilibrium of pay and working hours is likely to be a major impediment to redressing geographic imbalances in the distribution of health workers.

The low-level equilibrium of pay and working hours has led to an increase in the use of temporary contracts. In many cases this contradicts present norms and regulations. For example, temporary contracts are used to pay health workers holding permanent contracts for extra hours. Currently, approximately 10 percent of the wage bill is used to pay for staff members contracted temporarily. Actual use of health resources for paying staff members on temporary contracts is likely to be higher than this number indicates, because resources flowing from the national health insurance are used for the same purpose.

There is scope to improve the recruitment process. Current recruitment and transfer policies as well as the current incentive structure for health workers—salary, allowance schemes, and promotion and transfer policies—are not conducive to addressing geographic distribution and staff performance. This problem leads to inefficiencies in how wage bill resources are spent.

The recruitment process is supposed to be managed regionally but is still carried out mostly centrally. It is also heavily influenced by pressures from various professional associations and unions.

The system of transferring staff is complicated, involves many actors, and is not based on needs assessments in different geographic areas. However, transfers to the capital—which has one of the highest staff per population ratios—are banned.

Salaries vary widely among individuals with similar responsibilities and from region to region, which is in contrast to the stated policy that salaries are to be determined by job characteristics. Labor unions play a large role in setting salary levels.

Allowances can be used more strategically. Approximately 15 percent of the wage bill is spent on allowances. However, the system is complex and does not provide incentives to address the major challenges of imbalances in geographic distribution, low productivity, and poor quality of care. Labor unions also heavily influence the use of allowances.

Sanctioning, promotion, and transfer practices are not carried out according to policy. They do not provide incentives for good performance.

Notes

1. Note that these numbers are for SESPAS only and not total government health expenditure.
2. This information has not yet been published and is still in the evaluation process at SESPAS.

References

Albizu, Héctor, Temístocles Montás, and Vicente Bengoa. 2005. "Dominican Republic: Letter of Intent, Memorandum of Economic and Financial Policies, and Technical Memorandum of Understanding." International Monetary Fund, Washington, DC. http://www.imf.org/external/np/loi/2005/dom/011405.pdf.

———. 2006. "Dominican Republic: Letter of Intent and Annex to the Technical Memorandum of Understanding." International Monetary Fund, Washington, DC. http://www.imf.org/external/np/loi/2006/dom/042406.pdf.

———. 2007. "Dominican Republic: Letter of Intent, Memorandum of Economic and Financial Policies, and Technical Memorandum of Understanding." International Monetary Fund, Washington, DC. http://www.imf.org/external/np/loi/2007/dom/013107.pdf.

Chen, Lincoln, Timothy Evans, Sudhir Anand, Jo Ivey Boufford, Hilary Brown, Mushtaque Chowdhury, Marcos Cueto, Lola Dare, Gilles Dussault, Gijs Elzinga, Elizabeth Fee, Demissie Habte, Piya Hanvoravongchai, Marian Jacobs, Christoph Kurkowski, Sarah Michael, Ariel Pablos-Mendez, Nelson Sewankambo, Giorgio Solimano, Barbara Stilwell, Alex de Waal, and Suwit Wibulpolprasert. 2004. "Human Resources for Health: Overcoming the Crisis." *Lancet* 364 (9449): 1984–90.

Fedelino, Annalisa, Gerd Schwartz, and Marijn Verhoeven. 2006. "Aid Scaling Up: Do Wage Bill Ceilings Stand in the Way?" IMF Working Paper 06/106, International Monetary Fund, Washington, DC. http://www.imf.org/external/pubs/ft/wp/2006/wp06106.pdf.

Ferrinho, Paulo, Wim Van Lerberghe, Inês Fronteira, Fátima Hipólito, and André Biscaia. 2004. "Dual Practice in the Health Sector: Review of the Evidence." *Human Resources for Health* 2: 14. http://www.human-resources-health.com/content/2/1/14.

Novick, Marta, and Carlos Rosales. 2006. *Challenges to the Management of Human Resources for Health, 2005–2015*. Washington, DC: Pan American Health Organization. http://www.observatoriorh.org/Lima/docs/DesafiosGestionHR_eng.pdf.

OPS (Organización Panamericana de la Salud). 2007. "Perfil de los sistemas de salud de la República Dominicana: Monitoreo y análisis de los procesos de cambio y reforma." 3rd ed. OPS, Washington, DC.

Ribando, Clare M. 2005. "Dominican Republic: Political and Economic Conditions and Relations with the United States." CRS Report for Congress, Congressional Research Service, Library of Congress, Washington, DC. http://fpc.state.gov/documents/organization/46402.pdf.

World Bank. 2007. *World Development Indicators 2007*. Washington, DC: World Bank.

Comparative Analysis of Health Outcomes, Service Delivery, and Health Workforce Levels in Kenya, Zambia, Rwanda, and the Dominican Republic

Public Sector Provision of Health Services

In the four countries, the majority of people who sought treatment for fever, acute respiratory infection, or diarrhea did so in a public facility (table A.1).[1] Furthermore, between 65 percent and 91 percent of all deliveries in facilities occurred in the public sector. These statistics reveal the importance of the public sector in the provision of health care services. Because of data constraints, the actual proportion of health workers employed in the private and public sectors for these four countries is known only in Rwanda. But given the prominence of the public sector and the fact that in developing countries health workers who provide services in the private sector are often also employed in the public sector (Ferrinho and others 2004), the majority of the health workforce likely works in the public sector.

Table A.1   Share of Health Services Provided in the Public Sector

	Share (%)						
Type of service	Dominican Republic (2002)	Kenya (2003)	Rwanda (2000)	Zambia (2001)	Latin America average[a]	Sub-Saharan African average	Global average
Treatment of fever in a public facility	75	63	93	82	76	78	72
Medical treatment of acute respiratory infection	77	65	91	85	80	79	72
Medical treatment of diarrhea	77	68	95	83	78	80	72
Delivery in a facility	78	65	91	79	85	86	84

Source: Gwatkin and others 2007.
a. Latin American countries are Bolivia (1998 and 2003), Brazil (1996), Colombia (1995, 2000, and 2005), the Dominican Republic (1996 and 2002), Guatemala (1995 and 1999), Haiti (1995 and 2000), Nicaragua (1998 and 2001), Paraguay (1990), and Peru (1996 and 2000).

Analysis of Health Outcomes

As shown in table A.2, the infant mortality and maternal mortality rates in the Dominican Republic are better than the global average and close to or above those of Latin America. Kenya's outcomes are better than the average for Sub-Saharan Africa, while Rwanda's and Zambia's are well below the regional and global averages.

Figure A.1, however, shows that all four countries have above-average infant mortality and maternal mortality rates relative to gross domestic product and health spending per capita. In other words, other countries with similar per capita health spending and income levels experience better health outcomes.

Analysis of Health Service Delivery

At 98 percent, an above average figure for Latin America, the Dominican Republic has extremely high coverage of births attended by skilled health personnel (table A.2). Coverage rates in Kenya, Rwanda, and Zambia are all below the average for Sub-Saharan Africa. The Dominican Republic has

Table A.2   Outcome Indicators, 2005

Indicator	Dominican Republic	Kenya	Rwanda	Zambia	Latin America	Sub-Saharan Africa[a]	Global[a]
Infant mortality rate (deaths per 1,000 live births)	26	79	118	102	22	91	39
Maternal mortality rate (deaths per 100,000 live births)	150	560	1,300	830	149	829	304
Births attended by skilled health personnel (per 1,000 live births)[b]	98	42	35	43	89	54	79
DPT3 immunization rate (% of children 12–23 months)	77	76	95	80	90	74	87

Source: World Bank 2005.
a. Mean.
b. Mean of available data from 2000 to 2005.

above-average coverage of skilled birth attendance relative to income and health spending, whereas the three Sub-Saharan countries all fare worse than average (figure A.2).

In the case of DPT3 immunization rates, Rwanda far exceeds the average globally and regionally, as well as relative to its income and health spending levels. The presence of vertical programming for immunization in Rwanda may partially explain this outcome. Immunization rates in Kenya and Zambia are close to the global average, above the average for Sub-Saharan Africa, and close to the average relative to health spending and income. Rates in the Dominican Republic are below average relative to income and spending levels as well as when compared with those of other countries in the region.

Analysis of Health Workforce Levels

Table A.3 provides data on the total number of doctors and of all health workers for the public and private sectors combined. These data show the relative size of the health workforce and provide some interesting insights.[2] The Dominican Republic has slightly more health workers in relation to the regional average and relative to income and health

202

Figure A.1   Outcomes Relative to Income and Health Spending, 2005

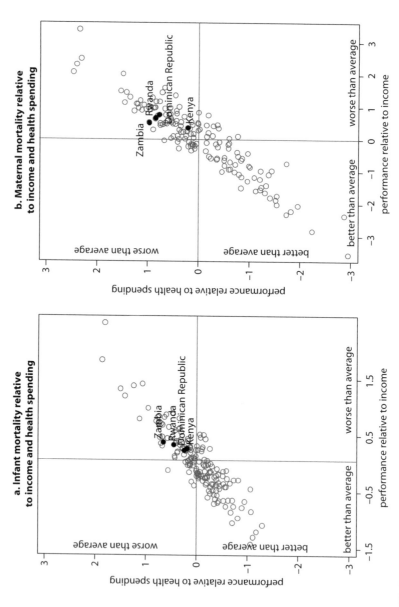

Source: World Bank 2007.

Figure A.2   Service Delivery Relative to Income and Health Spending, 2005

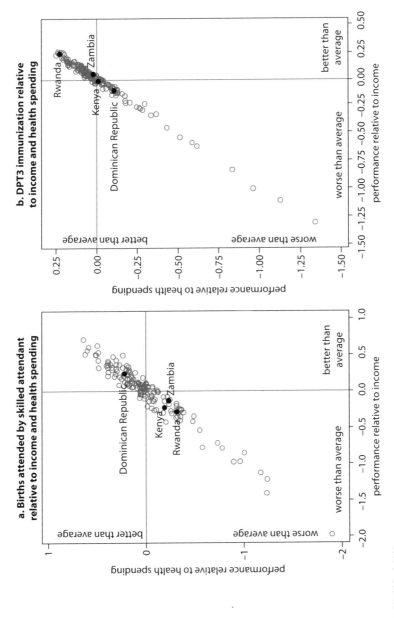

a. Births attended by skilled attendant relative to income and health spending

b. DPT3 immunization relative to income and health spending

Source: World Bank 2007.

Table A.3   Input Indicators, 2005

Indicator	Dominican Republic	Kenya	Rwanda	Zambia	Latin America	Sub-Saharan Africa[a]	Global[a]
Health workers per 1,000 population	4.96	2.05	2.06	2.8	4.53	2.34	6.50
Doctors per 1,000 population	1.88	0.14	0.05	0.12	1.44	0.20	1.44

Source: World Health Organization.
a. Mean.

spending (figure A.3). However, the number of doctors (while slightly higher than the regional average) is above average relative to income and health spending. Kenya, Zambia, and Rwanda also have a relatively high number of health workers but a relatively low number of doctors. The skill mix in these three countries is clearly less toward doctors and more toward other health care workers.

Summary and Key Points

In sum, this analysis suggests several important issues regarding how wage bill resources are used in the four countries. In Rwanda, Kenya, and Zambia, health outcomes and service delivery coverage are both below average. Underuse of services might partly explain the poor health outcomes. Interestingly, use is low despite the total number of health workers being high. With respect to workforce policy, this finding suggests a potential skill mix issue (supported by the fact that there are few doctors) or a geographic distribution, productivity, or quality of care issue. In the Dominican Republic, health outcomes are below average despite very high health service coverage. This finding suggests a quality of care rather than access issue. Interestingly, the skill mix in the Dominican Republic is skewed toward doctors, suggesting that with respect to workforce policy, the main issues could relate to productivity and quality of care—not geographic distribution or skill mix.

The analysis suggests that there are important issues in all four countries that are related to the management of the health wage bill. Moreover, the data suggest the issues are diverse and vary across countries. The analysis is meant to raise issues and to motivate the comprehensive work carried out in the specific case studies. It is not intended to draw a direct causal link between public sector wage bill management and health outcomes or

Figure A.3   Health Workforce Levels Relative to Health Spending and Income, 2005

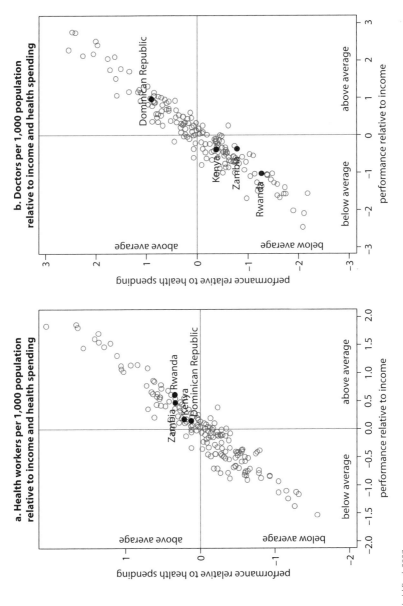

Source: World Bank 2007.

service delivery. Health outcomes can be attributed to a variety of issues beyond the health workforce and outside the health sector itself. These issues include access to water and sanitation, infrastructure, cultural and societal norms, educational attainment, and literacy. Because the public sector plays a pivotal role in the provision of health services, however, the manner in which the health wage bill is funded, allocated, and implemented is likely to have an important effect throughout the health system.

Notes

1. Treatment in a public facility includes treatment in (a) government hospitals, health centers, health posts, or dispensaries or (b) in facilities operated by government-affiliated social security programs. Total treatment figures do not include treatment obtained in private pharmacies or shops or from traditional healers. In some cases (Zambia), health workers are contracted out to private nonprofit organizations by the government; therefore, this government funding is not captured by the figures on treatment in a public facility.

2. The data in table A.3 are from the World Health Organization (WHO) and are quite consistent with the data collected in the country case studies. Small differences in some particular values, however, exist because of several factors, including year of data. For consistency and for comparison to regional and global averages, the WHO data are used in this table.

References

Ferrinho, Paulo, Wim Van Lerberghe, Inês Fronteira, Fátima Hipólito, and André Biscaia. 2004. "Dual Practice in the Health Sector: Review of the Evidence." *Human Resources for Health* 2: 14. http://www.human-resources-health.com/content/2/1/14.

Gwatkin, Davidson R., Shea Rutstein, Kiersten Johnson, Eldaw Suliman, Adam Wagstaff, and Agbessi Amouzou. 2007. *Socio-economic Differences in Health, Nutrition, and Population within Developing Countries.* Washington, DC: World Bank.

World Bank. 2005. *World Development Indicators 2005.* Washington, DC: World Bank.

———. 2007. *World Development Indicators 2007.* Washington, DC: World Bank.

Analysis of the Share of Government Health Expenditure Going to the Health Wage Bill: Some Stylized Facts

The share of government health expenditure devoted to paying health workers varies considerably across countries, ranging from below 10 percent to above 80 percent. Even within a country over time, considerable variation often occurs. Why would the ratio of wage to nonwage expenditure vary so much across countries? This appendix presents some stylized facts and potential hypotheses. It is meant to motivate further research rather than to provide clear conclusions.

There is a weak positive relationship between the share of government health expenditure going to the wage bill and health spending. A weak positive relationship also exists between the share of expenditure going to the wage bill and the gross domestic product (GDP). Governments in richer countries, on average, devote a slightly higher share of their health expenditure to the health wage bill (figures B.1 and B.2). The positive relationship may be for several reasons. The price ratio of labor to nonlabor inputs (for example, the ratio of wages of health workers to prices of pharmaceuticals or medical equipment) might be higher in wealthier countries (Nuxoll 1994). Insufficient cross-country data on wages of

Figure B.1   Health Wage Bill versus Income: Average, 2000–04

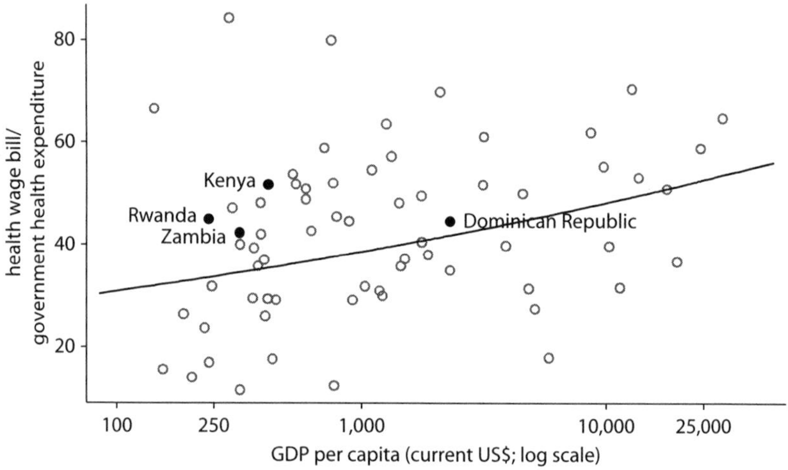

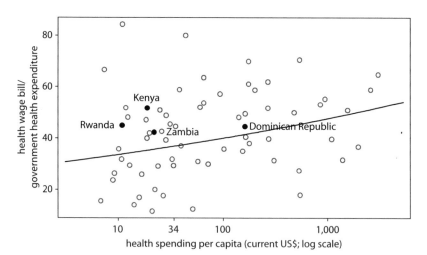

Source: World Bank 2007; World Health Organization.

Figure B.2   Health Wage Bill versus Health Spending: Average, 2000–04

Source: World Bank 2007; World Health Organization.

health workers exist to carry out such an analysis. It could also be that as health spending increases, countries may shift to a more expensive skill mix of health workers (that is, more doctors and fewer nurses) and, as a result, may need to shift more resources to wages.[1] It could also be that the production function for delivering health services may shift as health systems develop and health spending grows.[2]

Tremendous variation also occurs in the share of government health spending going to the wage bill across countries with similar health spending levels. This finding might be explained by differences in staffing levels, skill mix, price ratios, and production function for health services. In turn, for a given spending level, the production function (that is, the use of labor versus nonlabor inputs) may vary across countries because of differences in labor productivity. Countries with high labor productivity may not need as many health workers per bed or per pill to deliver services.

Only the analysis related to staffing levels and skill mix was carried out. The conclusion is that differences in overall staffing levels and skill mix do not fully explain the variation across countries with similar health spending levels. Controlling for health spending levels through regression analysis, one finds that countries that spend a higher share on the health wage bill do not systematically have a higher skill mix of staff (that is, more doctors relative to other health workers).

The share of government health expenditure devoted to the wage bill varies considerably by region (panel a, figure B.3). This finding is by far the most significant explanatory variable. The Latin American and Caribbean region has on average the highest share of government spending devoted to the health wage bill, and East Asia and the Pacific has the lowest. Variation also occurs across income group, as previously noted, with low-income countries at slightly lower levels on average (panel b, figure B.3). Similar to the preceding analysis, three factors might account for the regional variation: (a) differences in skill mix across regions, (b) differences in labor productivity across regions, and (c) differences in the ways that health workers are employed in the public sector across regions.

The region with the highest share of government health spending devoted to the wage bill (Latin America and the Caribbean) also has the highest use of doctors, who tend to be the most expensive type of health worker to employ (analysis not shown). No standard measures of workforce productivity exist, but dual practice and absenteeism are common features in many developing countries across all regions (Novick and Rosales 2006). Thus, the regional analysis supports some of the hypotheses that are not supported by the cross-country analysis.

The way health workers are employed and paid in the public sector is likely to affect significantly the share of government health expenditure devoted to the wage bill. In some countries, health workers in the public sector are employed by the government as part of either a national or a

Figure B.3   Health Sector Wage Bill as a Share of Public Spending on Health, Mean 2000–04

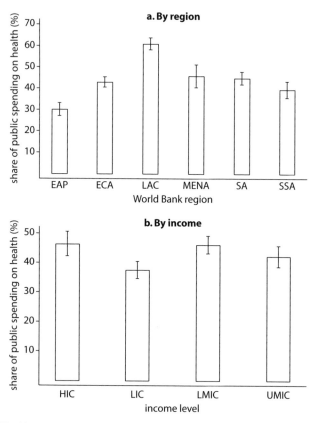

Source: World Health Organization.

Note: EAP = East Asia and the Pacific; ECA = Europe and Central Asia; LAC = Latin America and the Caribbean; MENA = Middle East and North Africa; SA = South Asia; SSA = Sub-Saharan Africa; HIC = high-income countries; LIC = low-income countries; LMIC = low- and middle-income countries; UMIC = upper-middle-income countries.

subnational civil service. In other countries, health workers in the public sector are employed by facilities, and their wages are paid from the operating budgets that are received as transfers from the central or provincial governments. In the latter case, wages paid to health workers are not a separate item in the government accounts but are part of transfers to service providers. Therefore, in countries where health service delivery is highly decentralized, one would expect the share of government health expenditure going to wages to be low. Few adequate cross-country indicators measure the level of health service decentralization. However, because East Asia and the Pacific, the region that tends to have the highest level of decentralization of service delivery (Green 2005), also has the lowest share of health spending devoted to the wage bill, this explanation seems at least plausible.

A weak negative relationship exists between the share of government health expenditure devoted to the wage bill and the level of donor assistance (figure B.4). Donors in the health sector have traditionally not funded recurrent salary costs of health workers unless indirectly through budget support. If donor assistance for health is concentrated on non-labor inputs and governments coordinate well with donors in planning expenditures, then governments in countries receiving high donor aid might devote more health expenditure to the wage bill. Alternatively, if government health expenditure is not well coordinated with donor activity, there might be no relationship. The analysis, however, shows a slightly negative relationship. This outcome suggests some other country-level factor that might drive both donor funding levels and the share of government health expenditure devoted to the wage bill. The modality of donor funding—whether it is general budget support, stand-alone programs, or sectorwide approaches—is also likely to affect the relationship, but this effect was not examined.

Examining trends over time within a sample of countries can be useful to control for country-level fixed effects. The data for Ghana indeed

Figure B.4   Health Wage Bill versus External Resources for Health, Average 2000–04

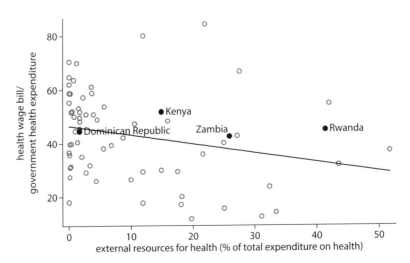

Source: World Bank 2007; World Health Organization.

suggest that the government is shifting its expenditure toward salaries and allowances (personnel emoluments and additional duty hours allowance in figure B.5), and donors are funding nonsalary items. This trend has resulted in a situation where over 90 percent of government health expenditure is going to the wage bill.

Figure B.5   Distribution of Government and Donor Health Expenditure in Ghana, 1999–2005

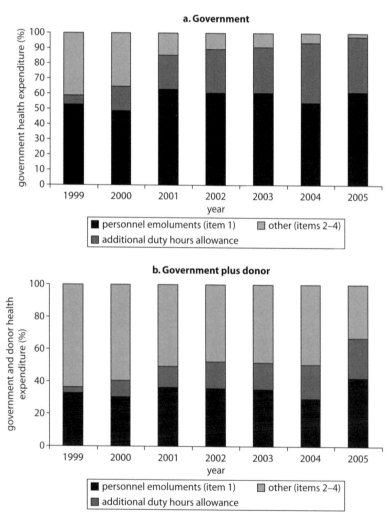

Source: Ghana Ministry of Health.

Figure B.6   Health Wage Bill as a Share of Government Health Expenditure in Two Regions, 1998–2004

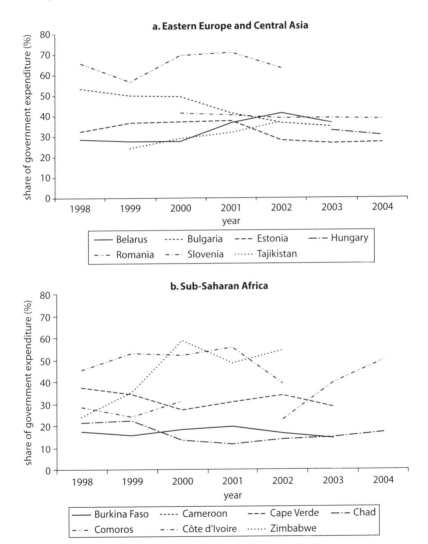

Source: World Health Organization.

The share of health spending devoted to the wage bill is fairly stable overall but can be quite volatile in some countries. The average across countries in the standard deviation over time is only 4.6 percentage points. However, this standard deviation varies from 1.1 percentage points in Mongolia to 14.2 percentage points in Kenya. The highest volatility was in Sub-Saharan Africa, which had a standard deviation of 5.7 percentage points compared with about 3.5 percentage points in all the other regions (figure B.6).

Notes

1. Cross-country data analysis shows a very weak relationship between health spending levels and the ratios of doctors to other health workers, suggesting that this hypothesis is not supported by the data.

2. If anything, however, this scenario would result in a negative relationship between health spending and the share of health spending going to the wage bill. A stethoscope and a medical officer may be the first unit of health service delivery as countries develop. As countries grow and more and more sophisticated health services are provided, more nonlabor inputs, such as equipment and pharmaceuticals, are incorporated into the production function.

References

Green, Amanda E. 2005. "Managing Human Resources in a Decentralized Context." In *East Asia Decentralizes, Making Local Government Work*, 129–53. Washington, DC: World Bank. http://siteresources.worldbank.org/INTEAPDECEN/Resources/Chapter-7.pdf.

Novick, Marta, and Carlos Rosales. 2006. *Challenges to the Management of Human Resources for Health, 2005–2015*. Washington, DC: Pan American Health Organization. http://www.observatoriorh.org/Lima/docs/DesafiosGestionHR_eng.pdf.

Nuxoll, Daniel A. 1994. "Differences in Relative Prices and International Differences in Growth Rates." *American Economic Review* 84 (5): 1423–36.

World Bank. 2007. *World Development Indicators 2007*. Washington, DC: World Bank.

Decentralization and Human Resources for Health

In the country case studies examined as part of this report as well as in other developing countries, several sources of inefficiency exist in the public sector in the way wage bill resources are used in the health sector. The main categories are administrative efficiency (for example, whether the wage bill budget is executed fully or the recruitment process is timely) and allocative efficiency (for example, whether additional wage bill resources are allocated to areas where staff are needed most and whether the remuneration policies and terms of work provide incentives for retention in underserved areas, low absenteeism, high productivity, and quality of care). In the country case studies, one major driver of inefficiency found was the high degree of centralization of human resources for health (HRH) management functions, coupled with low capacity in central agencies. One policy option to address this issue is to decentralize key HRH functions to subnational units such as provinces, districts, and facilities. This appendix summarizes the rationale behind decentralizing key functions and the available evidence and lessons learned about its effect.

Decentralization refers to transferring decision-making authority to subnational levels. It is a term that has many meanings, and distinguishing

---

This appendix was prepared by Andrew Mitchell with input from the core team.

among different types of decentralization is important. Decentralization can be defined as the transfer of authorities from central government bodies to lower levels within the public sector or to autonomous institutions (Rondinelli, Nellis, and Cheema 1984). Decentralization is often categorized along political, fiscal, and administrative lines. Political decentralization extends decision-making power governing public institutions to citizens at the local level. Fiscal decentralization relates to subnational ability to control financial resources, including revenue generation and allocation of funds. Administrative decentralization refers to relationships of authority that affect the managerial concerns. Often viewed along a continuum of lesser and greater degrees of decentralization, administrative decentralization may be characterized as *deconcentration* of authorities from the central to local levels within a ministry or department of health, *delegation* of authorities to semiautonomous bodies, and *devolution* of responsibilities to autonomous or separate local governments (Hutchinson and LaFond 2004).

In general, political, fiscal, and administrative decentralization may be applied to any number of distinct functions in the health sector. A ministry or department of health oversees several kinds of health functions, including those that relate to financing of services (for example, expenditures allocation); service organization (for example, provider payment mechanisms); governance (for example, facility oversight boards); and human resources (Bossert 1998). Decentralization within one function, such as financing for services through block grants, does not necessarily imply decentralization within other functions, such as ability to modify centrally determined program priorities. Indeed, human resource functions are often among the least decentralized, likely because of the large share (and therefore control) of the health sector budget generally allocated to personnel (Bossert and Beauvais 2002). In Ghana, for instance, despite devolution of provision of primary health care and complete delinking of health providers from the Ministry of Health, human resource functions remain highly centralized (Dovlo 1998).

Rationale for Decentralization

There is strong rationale for transferring decision making to subnational units as a means of improving efficiency of expenditure in the public sector. The rationale behind decentralization is relatively straightforward: smaller organizations that operate with autonomy and close to their clients are generally more agile, innovative, and responsive to local needs than large, centralized organizations (Saltman, Bankauskaite, and Vrangbaek

2007). More proximity between health sector decision makers and catchment populations, for instance, can better orient service provision to local health priorities and therefore increase use of and satisfaction with health services. Decentralized units with greater autonomy may also more innovatively face challenges in HRH financing, allocation, and management. Table C.1 summarizes common objectives of decentralization, the mechanisms by which decentralization may achieve those objectives, and reasons that decentralization might not meet objectives.

In the area of HRH, decentralization can mean many different things. It is important to distinguish which particular decision-making powers are transferred to local authorities. Table C.2 lists the major human resource functions that might be decentralized independently or in concert. They include functions related to employment (hiring and firing, nature of tenure, defining the compensation package); management (transfers, promotions, and sanctions); skills mix; and training. Transferring authority to the local level for these functions may help governments be more responsive to local conditions, including market conditions, citizen preferences, patient needs, staff availability, and available resources.

There is a strong rationale for why transferring certain functions to local units might improve administrative and allocative efficiency, but potential negative effects also exist. In terms of administrative efficiency, allowing local recruitment could shorten the time to fill a position, eliminating the many steps involved with central-level approval. It may also lead to a better match of candidates with the appropriate

Table C.1   Rationales for Decentralization

Objective	Mechanism	Potential drawbacks
Improved administrative efficiency	• Less bureaucratic red tape and more experimentation • Greater local-level cost consciousness	• Higher national-level transaction costs from local-level administrative redundancies
Improved allocative efficiency	• Greater responsiveness to local-level priorities and preferences	• Heightened inequities at the national level
Greater accountability	• Heightened local-level involvement and civic participation	• Minimum level of local-level capacity required • Open to local-level capture
Improved quality of services	• Improvements in efficiency and accountability • Greater innovation from increased autonomy	• All of the above

Source: Authors' compilation.

Table C.2   Decentralization of Human Resource Functions

Function	Specific elements	Rationale for decentralization
Hiring and firing	• Selection of candidates, development of job descriptions, and termination of staff members	• Reduces time to fill vacant positions • Matches candidates to job profiles better
Tenure	• Determination of terms of employment (for example, permanent versus contracted staff members)	• Responds to local market conditions • Allows more flexibility in types of personnel hired
Salary	• Determination of base salary	• Responds to local market conditions in recruiting health workers
Nonsalary compensation	• Determination of allowances, bonuses, and pensions	• Responds to local market conditions in recruiting health workers
Transfers	• Transfer of staff members within and between localities • Horizontal mobility	• Increases flexibility in deploying staff members • Responds to local preferences, patient needs, and staff availability
Promotions and sanctioning	• Promotion, performance review, grievances, and termination	• Makes promotions more timely
Skills mix	• Determination of overall staff establishment • Determination of facility staffing patterns • Accreditation and licensing standards	• Responds to local market conditions, local preferences, patient needs, staff availability, and staffing resources
Training	• Central or local division of preservice and in-service training responsibilities	• Responds to local preferences, patient needs, staff availability, and staffing resources

Source: Authors' compilation

position, because the final selection of candidates would be done locally. The same holds for firing, because dismissal and sanctioning could be conducted much more quickly. Similarly, letting local units set salaries and allowances allows them to take into account local labor market conditions. For example, salaries for certain areas may need to be much higher to attract staff members, but common national pay scales may prevent such local discretion. However, these potential gains in efficiency are threatened by negative repercussions if proper oversight and monitoring are not in place. Allowing local hiring and firing may increase the likelihood of corruption and nepotism, as has been reported in China, Indonesia, Tanzania, and Uganda (for example, favoritism in employment toward "sons and daughters of the soil," a form of nepotism) (Ssengooba 2005; Tang and Bloom 2000; Turner and others 2003). Decentralizing wage-setting could exacerbate distributional inequities if historically advantaged localities are better able to attract and retain personnel than are relatively disadvantaged areas. It might also lead to wage inflation as districts and provinces compete for scarce personnel and escalation in the overall wage bill if controls are lacking or not all local-level workers are under local contracts (a common occurrence). This has been the experience of such countries as the Philippines and Mexico, where local government units have felt fiscal pressure to raise compensation of locally employed personnel to the higher pay scales enjoyed by workers who continue to be centrally employed (Homedes and Ugalde 2005; World Bank and Asian Development Bank 2005).

For decentralization to work, careful thought must be given to what functions need to be matched. For example, transferring authority to hire and fire workers may have less of an effect if authority on setting the skill mix is not transferred as well (that is, the local government may be able to select which individual to hire but not whether to hire a doctor or a nurse because of fixed staffing norms). Authority to set salaries might not be useful unless either facilities have flexibility in how much of their budget can be used to pay health workers, or facility budgets are adjusted based on local salary levels. In other words, an appropriate match needs to be made between fiscal and administrative functions.

Decentralization in Practice

The scope of decentralization of HRH functions has been limited in developing countries. Although examples exist of countries that have undergone a process of human resource decentralization, governments often decentralize only some elements of certain human resource functions. Under less expansive forms of decentralization (for example, deconcentration or delegation), the most commonly decentralized functions appear to relate to human resource management, whereas functions related to terms of employment for HRH (for example, determination of local-level wage bill or HRH salaries) tend to remain under centralized control. Furthermore, the degree of decentralization within a specific functional element can vary. In Tanzania, for example, recruitment and selection procedures for junior staff fall under district-level auspices while the same functions for senior-level staff remain centralized. Even under more expansive forms of decentralization (for example, devolution), salary determination may be specifically delinked from the decentralization process to ensure continued central control, as is the case in the Philippines. Public sector decentralization experiences in East Asia are typical of this pattern. Among the six countries analyzed (Cambodia, China, Indonesia, the Philippines, Thailand, and Vietnam), none is able to determine salaries at the local level (though top-ups are allowed), whereas all but one handle recruitment at the local level (Green 2005: ix, 135).

For many administrative, political, and policy-related reasons, most countries have limited the scope of decentralization of HRH functions. Administratively, a "big bang" approach to decentralization of HRH functions is costly and may require fundamental organizational changes of national health ministries. Terms of employment and terms of reference for posts—existing and planned—may need to be redesigned to incorporate new administrative responsibilities, skill requirements, and resources available at different levels of the system. Although such reform was possible in a country such as Indonesia, which has a highly capable civil service commission at the national level, such capacities may not exist elsewhere. Even where they do, the financial implications of decentralization can be significant: Mexico spent an estimated US$452 million in administrative costs to transfer its federal health employees to the state level (Homedes and Ugalde 2005).

The required local-level capacity to implement these changes might be lacking and cause hesitation to decentralize human resource functions. Indeed, the quality of Papua New Guinea's personnel management database rapidly deteriorated following provincial-level devolution (Kolehmainen-Aitken 2001). Additionally, the associated costs of ensuring that newly decentralized systems work efficiently could be exorbitant and meet with resistance. Chief executives of local governments in the Philippines, for example, initially refused to absorb over 4 percent of devolved health staff (Kolehmainen-Aitken 2001).

Political pressure may prevent decentralization. Politically, human resource decentralization involves a wide variety of institutional actors, both within the government (for example, health managers, civil service officials, elected politicians) and in the private sector (for example, professional associations, unions). These stakeholders may manifest resistance to decentralization of HRH functions for any number of reasons. Bolivia, for example, has twice failed to decentralize HRH functions despite fiscal decentralization because of resistance both from within the government and from most unions and professional associations (World Bank 2004). Similar resistance has been manifested in Burkina Faso (Bodart and others 2001) and elsewhere. Furthermore, ministries of health often do not have the ability to alter key HRH functions such as civil service–wide terms of employment.

Finally, central authorities may limit decentralization of human resource functions in light of certain policy objectives. Although decentralization may improve local-level responsiveness to needs, it may neglect national-level concerns, such as equity in HRH distribution or standards of compensation. In Uganda, for instance, district governments must adhere to a national pay scale even if benefits and allowances are left to their discretion (Bossert and Beauvais 2002). The government explicitly developed this system to ensure equity in deployment of personnel among local governments (Ssengooba 2005). In Brazil, an important federally supported primary health care program specifically retains many staffing concerns (for example, composition of teams, personnel job descriptions) even while program implementation has been devolved to the municipal level. This design was reportedly used specifically to ensure that local implementation met national objectives as well as to avoid political program capture (Guanais de Aguiar 2006).

Evidence of the Impact of Decentralization

What does the evidence say? The following evidence is informed by a literature review, conducted in March and April 2008. Documents consulted include peer-reviewed journal articles; other published works (for example, books, official reports); and public domain "gray literature" (that is, unpublished or nonreviewed literature). All sources or relevant citations were accessed over the Internet. Primary search engines included PubMed (for peer-reviewed sources), Google (for gray literature), and site-specific searches (for example, USAID Development Experience Clearinghouse). Manual searches of bibliographic references contained within the documents retrieved were also made to identify further instances of relevant literature. The research strategy was not designed as a reproducible systematic review of the literature.

Discussion of the evidence base focuses primarily on links between decentralization of management-oriented human resource functions and efficiency or performance. Although insights on the role that decentralized salary determination might play in these outcomes is of great interest, the general lack of experience with decentralization of salary setting in developing countries precludes such an analysis.

Improved administrative efficiency is context-specific and requires adequate capacity at local levels. Instances exist in which decentralization of hiring and firing appears to improve administrative efficiency. Delegation of recruitment procedures in Thailand from the central civil service commission to line ministries is reported to have reduced this process by over 50 percent—from 68 to 31 days (Simananta and Aramkul n.d.). In China, devolution to the township level of recruitment for health facility personnel enabled health centers to better match demand with supply costs and to reduce employment by 70 percent (Liu and others 2006). In Uganda, three-quarters of health workers interviewed in one study felt that salary disbursement is more rapid following district-level decentralization of human resource functions related to recruitment, selection, performance evaluation, and promotion (Ssengooba 2005; also box C.1). In other instances, however, drawbacks to decentralization

---

Box C.1

A Tale of Two Ugandas: Successes and Failures in Administrative Efficiency under Decentralized Human Resource Management

The framework of decentralization of human resource functions in Uganda is typical of that of many countries. Most human resource management functions—recruitment, appointment, allowance and benefit setting, performance evaluation, and promotion—are under the authority of district service commissions (DSCs), whereas salary scales and payroll management remain under centralized control by the Ministry of Public Service. Before this decentralized framework, administrative inefficiencies clearly abounded in human resource management. Many employees worked without ever receiving formal letters of appointment, for example, while others remained indefinitely on probation for no apparent reasons. Decentralization has been able to address some of these problems, but challenges remain.

Successes

Interviews with 800 health workers carried out in 2005 suggest that, in many ways, decentralization has improved human resource management:

(continued)

- Under demand-driven recruitment, employment processes are generally much faster, owing to the ability of DSCs to conduct selection. Furthermore, decentralized recruitment may have allowed districts to better match needs with resources: poorer districts generally had higher levels of workers working in their home district than did wealthier districts.
- Around half of study respondents felt that performance appraisals were more objective after decentralization than previously, and most felt that heightened local-level supervision and accountability were beneficial.
- Almost three-quarters of respondents receive salaries more quickly under decentralization and expressed satisfaction that, under decentralization, the date of monthly payments was simply predictable.
- District facilities were able to employ some cadres of personnel at significantly higher rates than nationally established minimum staffing standards.

Failures

For each success, there is a flip side. Additionally, decentralization of human resource management has introduced new challenges not of previous concern:

- The change from centralized supply-driven recruitment to decentralized demand-driven recruitment—coupled with broader national-level policies to contain the public sector wage bill (wage ceiling; freeze on recruitment)—left many job seekers feeling frustrated about not being able to find employment. Although some districts increased the level of locally employed workers, this action may have been driven by nepotism as much as by taking advantage of market conditions. Health workers working in their home districts generally reported expedient recruitment, whereas those from other home districts often perceived the recruitment process as biased against them.
- Though performance evaluations are more objective, many respondents felt that these evaluations were not used in employment and promotion decisions. Furthermore, 75 percent of respondents did not feel secure in their jobs because of the power of local authorities to dismiss workers and the perception that these authorities often base employment decisions on nontechnical or non-job-related grounds.
- Although satisfaction has increased with more efficient salary disbursement, it is in some ways overshadowed by low salary levels: for only one in five respondents does salary make up even one-half of total earnings; the remainder comes from subsistence cultivation, private practice, other business, and the like.

(continued)

Box C.1 *(Continued)*

- Employees expressed a widespread sense of entrapment because of new obstacles to cross-district transfer under decentralization. (Workers effectively have to resign from their post in one district before taking another job in a different district.)
- Employment of health workers above minimum standards was confined almost exclusively to nontechnical personnel. For technical personnel, shortfalls from minimum standards ranged from 25 to 50 percent.

Lessons Learned

Uganda's experience with decentralization and HRH provides useful insights to countries considering decentralization of human resource functions. Uganda's successes and failures suggest that to achieve improvements in administrative efficiency under decentralization, the following conditions should apply:

- Adequate local capacity and accountability need to accompany increased local-level authority. Heightened efficiency in recruitment means little if overall salary levels are not adequate to attract and retain workers. Accountability can be effective, but only if it is not subject to local political capture.
- An appropriate balance must be struck between degrees of decentralization and centralization. Although local and demand-driven recruitment is in some ways more efficient than centralized and supply-driven recruitment, the absence of centralized coordination of information about job availability—as well as new obstacles to cross-district transfers and promotions—has resulted in an expensive system for job seekers and an entrapping system for workers.
- Effectiveness of HR decentralization is greatly affected by broader constraints. Financial limitations imposed by national-level policies to contain the country's civil service wage bill became the overriding criterion for determining staffing patterns and inhibited the ability of DSCs to respond to local conditions.

Source: Ssengooba 2005.

described in table C.1 have prevented efficiency gains. District-level decentralization of certain human resource management functions in Pakistan is said to have resulted in long-term vacancies of posts, in part caused by multiple and overlapping lines of authority over posting of officials (Nayyar-Stone and others 2006). Despite decentralization of recruitment and contracting procedures in Tanzania to the district level for lower-level personnel, employment procedures remain lengthy, and delays in hiring continue as before. A lack of local-level awareness of procedures and inadequate financial resources are cited as contributory factors (Dominick and Kurowski 2004; Kimaro and Sahay 2004).

Decentralization generally does not narrow—or even accentuates—inequities in geographic distribution of personnel. Country experiences suggest that inabilities to guide the decentralization process with national-level objectives—as well as increased local-level transaction costs—inhibit equity in distribution of personnel. Geographic inequities in HRH distribution have been perpetuated where the central ministry of health no longer has the authority to establish staffing establishments (for example, China, Papua New Guinea) or the capacity to fulfill such establishments, despite decentralization of human resource management functions. For example, one-third of Mozambique's health facilities—for which selection, recruitment, posting, administrative procedures on salaries, and retirement are handled by provincial governors—do not meet nationally determined staffing patterns (Ferrinho and Omar 2006; Kolehmainen-Aitken and Shipp 1990; Tang and Bloom 2000). At the same time, increased bureaucratic hurdles at the local level can further perpetuate geographic imbalances. Devolution of human resource functions in Indonesia to provincial, regional, and city governments, for example, has not mitigated existing inequities in distribution (in the health sector, the ratio of HRH to 1,000 population ranges from 0.5 to 5.5 at the regional level, with one- to fivefold differences at the city or district level). The lack of a formal process to transfer staff members between regions—as well as no national downsizing plan to meet equity concerns—may help perpetuate these imbalances (Thabrany 2006; Turner and others 2003). Difficulties in transferring staff members between local governmental units endowed with devolved human resource powers have also been reported in China, Papua New Guinea, and Tanzania (Campos-Outcalt, Kewa, and Thomason 1995; Dominick and Kurowski 2004; Liu and others 2006). Additionally, HRH decentralization can heighten or even create horizontal inequities among personnel. Reports from China, the Philippines, and Uganda indicate that staff members who perform similar functions are paid differently because some continue to be administered centrally while others are paid locally (Kolehmainen-Aitken 2004).

Evidence on quality of care is scant, mixed, and of limited generalizability. On the quality side, a particularly interesting account from Tanzania suggests that decentralization of human resource functions is positively associated with quality of care. Analyzing the degree of decentralization in governmental and nongovernmental health facilities—measured by ability to fire personnel, set salary levels, pay workers from local resources, and determine staffing patterns—the author finds greater decentralization to be associated with better quality of care (including metrics on clinical and diagnostic procedures, health education, and client responsiveness) (Mliga 2003). Though provocative, this study is plagued with methodological limitations that make the influence of decentralization impossible to isolate from other factors (such as different quality of personnel by institution ownership type).

Similarly, little or conflicting evidence is available related to absenteeism or turnover. One study states that assumption of recruitment and appointment powers for contracted physicians by divisional-level authorities in Pakistan has reduced absenteeism (Collins, Omar, and Tarin 2002), although another indicates findings to the contrary (Nayyar-Stone and others 2006). In Nigeria, relatively elevated rates of facility turnover suggest that the national civil service incentive structure is not meeting its objectives of heightened facility-level teamwork and stability despite human resource management having been fully devolved to local governments (Das Gupta, Gauri, and Khemani 2004).

In summary, there are both success and failure stories in the literature, clearly showing no magic bullets are available for improving HRH performance through decentralization. Moreover, the evidence base is fairly weak. It is increasingly clear that health sector decentralization is not an automatic prescription for improved efficiency or performance. This applies equally to decentralization of human resource functions and to health functions more generally. Although connections may exist between decentralization of human resource functions and efficiency and performance, evidence from the previous literature is not strong. A major reason is a lack of research on the effect of decentralization on outcomes. This knowledge gap is particularly deep for outcomes related to administrative efficiency. Of the examples cited previously, only the China and Thailand accounts provide quantitative data to support their conclusions, making evaluation of the accuracy of claims made by these reports generally impossible. More generally, rigorously evaluating the effects of decentralization on administrative efficiency does not appear to be on anyone's agenda.

Even with more rigorous studies, a second reason has to do with the difficulty in attributing decentralization of human resource functions per se to outcomes. On the one hand, the multifaceted nature of decentralization makes isolating the effect of decentralizing any one element of a given function difficult. For instance, the precise role that decentralization of human resource functions has played in geographic distribution of

HRH—as opposed to other factors, such as the capacity of regions to effectively finance HRH under fiscal decentralization—is not documented. On the other hand, decentralization is almost always but one component of a larger package of health reforms, any of which might affect efficiency and quality concerns related to HRH. In China, for instance, loosening of HRH rural service requirement rules occurred at the same time that human resource management functions were devolved to townships. The subsequent reported increase in employment of "unskilled staff members" and suboptimal facility staffing patterns may have had as much to do with decreased incentives to locate in certain facilities as human resource management decentralization.

The evidence suggests several key issues that need to be considered in undertaking decentralization of human resource functions to achieve intended aims. At the local level, adequate capacity and accountability are key ingredients. Where decentralization has failed to meet desired goals, many previous studies have pointed to the lack of adequate financial resources made available to local authorities to carry out human resource functions as a major factor. In essence, decentralization of management functions cannot be expected to improve service delivery without accompanying ability to fund those functions. Similarly, several analyses point to lack of local-level accountability in thwarting goals of decentralization. In China, Indonesia, Tanzania, and Uganda, for example, favoritism in employment toward "sons and daughters of the soil" is reportedly common because of local political capture of the decentralization process (Ssengooba 2005; Tang and Bloom 2000; Turner and others 2003).

Both constraints and opportunities to effective human resource decentralization also exist at the national level. Constraints often come in the form of policies that supersede a country's national health policy-making body. Many of the countries analyzed have rigid civil service employment structures, have imposed wage ceilings, or are in the process of downsizing the public sector workforce. Such constraints may inherently inhibit the range of human resource functions that can be decentralized and thus the likely effect of decentralization. At the same time, a ministry of health or relevant policy-making body needs to take advantage of opportunities to steer the course of decentralization. First and foremost, clarity in the objectives and divisions of responsibilities under decentralization are prerequisites. Confusion in lines of authority is often cited as a challenge to effective human resource decentralization. Districts in Kenya, for instance, are expected to manage public sector HRH performance but are not legally granted this function (Steffensen and others 2004). Additionally, there is no reason to expect local-level authorities to develop innovative ways to improve efficiency or performance without national-level incentives to do so. The experience of primary health care in Nigeria—in which most local governments continue to abide by national civil service standards in setting pay rather than use performance or other locally relevant criteria—is a case in point (Das Gupta, Gauri, and Khemani 2004).

Key Messages

In summary, decentralizing human resource functions is a complex affair requiring a program of functional transfer of powers that matches national- and local-level capacities, resources, and accountability. When one is designing a program of human resource decentralization, considering the following points could help:

- *Objectives of human resource decentralization at the local and national levels need to be explicitly formulated and prioritized.* Given limited health sector budgets and capacities, it is doubtful that most countries will be able to register across-the-board improvements in efficiency and performance that could be realized under decentralization. Additionally, national-level priorities are not always in line with those at the local level. A program of human resource decentralization therefore needs to balance and prioritize local-level discretion in addressing the most pressing concerns at that level with national-level concerns.

- *Mechanisms by which human resource decentralization can achieve objectives need to be clearly articulated.* Decentralization is often thwarted by conflicting policies of centralization along one function, decentralization along another, lack of capacities to implement either, and lack of accountability to oversee implementation. In large part, this problem arises because objectives have not been clearly defined, nor have the tensions between local and national levels inherent in decentralization been addressed. Mapping out the mechanisms by which human resource decentralization is expected to meet objectives would go a long way toward developing more coherent and successful programs of decentralization. If improving administrative efficiency is the highest priority, for example, decentralizing management functions (for example, recruitment and selection) might be enough without necessarily decentralizing salary determination for those positions. If, however, such allocative efficiencies as inequitable geographic distribution dominate, giving lower levels greater authority in setting salaries to attract HRH to underserved areas might be more effective, whether recruitment or selection takes place at the central or peripheral levels. Similarly, although minimum national facility staffing standards may help to ensure equity in HRH distribution, they come at the expense of flexibility to adapt to local conditions. Whether such standards are worthwhile requires prioritizing objectives and thinking through which package of minimum standards will actually achieve those objectives.

- *Policy makers should address capacity constraints and create incentives in line with objectives.* Time and again, inadequate central-level support (technically, financially, administratively) has been cited as a major roadblock for effectively decentralizing human resource functions. A program of decentralization needs to be realistic about what gains can be expected, given existing capacities, as well as ways in which those capacities can be improved. Additionally, capacities may be necessary for human resource decentralization, but they are not necessarily sufficient. Incentives are needed to encourage local decision makers to make the most of opportunities afforded by greater control of human resource functions.

- *The effect of human resource decentralization on efficiency and performance needs to be monitored.* Improving the balance sheet of decentralization and HRH requires a much better understanding of the links between (a) human resource decentralization and (b) efficiency and performance. This understanding can be developed only through a concerted program of research to evaluate the effects of human resource decentralization on outcomes.

References

Bodart, Claude, Gérard Servais, Yansané L. Mohamed, and Bergis Schmidt-Ehry. 2001. "The Influence of Health Sector Reform and External Assistance in Burkina Faso." *Health Policy and Planning* 16 (1): 74–86.

Bossert, Thomas J. 1998. "Analyzing the Decentralization of Health Systems in Developing Countries: Decision Space, Innovation, and Performance." *Social Science and Medicine* 47 (10): 1513–27.

Bossert, Thomas J., and Joel C. Beauvais. 2002. "Decentralization of Health Systems in Ghana, Zambia, Uganda, and the Philippines: A Comparative Analysis of Decision Space." *Health Policy and Planning* 17 (1): 14–31.

Campos-Outcalt, Doug, Kelly Kewa, and Jane Thomason. 1995. "Decentralization of Health Services in Western Highlands Province, Papua New Guinea: An Attempt to Administer Health Service at the Subdistrict Level." *Social Science and Medicine* 40 (8): 1091–98.

Collins, C. D., Mayeh Omar, and Ehsanullah Tarin. 2002. "Decentralization, Health Care and Policy Process in the Punjab, Pakistan in the 1990s." *International Journal of Health Planning and Management* 17 (2): 123–46.

Das Gupta, Monica, Varun Gauri, and Stuti Khemani. 2004. "Decentralized Delivery of Primary Health Services in Nigeria: Survey Evidence from the States of Lagos and Kogi." Africa Region Human Development Working Paper, World Bank, Washington, DC.

Dominick, Anna, and Christoph Kurowski. 2004. *Human Resources for Health: An Appraisal of the Status Quo in Tanzania Mainland.* Washington, DC: World Bank.

Dovlo, Delanyo. 1998. "Health Sector Reform and Deployment, Training, and Motivation of Human Resources towards Equity in Health Care: Issues and Concerns in Ghana." Ministry of Health, Accra. http://www.hrhresourcecenter. org/node/181.

Ferrinho, Paulo, and Caroline Omar. 2006. "The Human Resources for Health Situation in Mozambique." Africa Region Human Development Working Paper 91, Human Development Sector, Africa Region, World Bank.

Green, Amanda. 2005. "Managing Human Resources in a Decentralized Context." In *East Asia Decentralizes, Making Local Government Work*, 129–53. Washington, DC: World Bank. http://siteresources.worldbank.org/INTEAPDE CEN/Resources/Chapter-7.pdf.

Guanais de Aguiar, Frederico Campos. 2006. "Evaluating the Health Impacts of Primary Care Decentralization in the Context of a Developing Country." PhD diss., New York University, New York.

Homedes, Núria, and Antonio Ugalde. 2005. "Human Resources: The Cinderella of Health Sector Reform in Latin America." *Human Resources for Health* 3 (1): 1.

Hutchinson, Paul L., and Anne K. LaFond. 2004. *Monitoring and Evaluation of Decentralization Reforms in Developing Country Health Sectors.* Bethesda, MD: Partners for Health Reform*plus* Project, Abt Associates.

Kimaro, Honest C., and Sundeep Sahay 2004. "An Institutional Perspective on the Process of Decentralization of Health Information Systems: A Case Study from Tanzania." *Information Technology for Development* 13 (4): 363–90.

Kolehmainen-Aitken, Riitta-Liisa. 2001. "Decentralization and Human Resources: Implications and Impact." *Human Resources Development Journal* 2: 1.

———. 2004. "Decentralization's Impact on the Health Workforce: Perspectives of Managers, Workers and National Leaders." *Human Resources for Health* 2 (1): 5.

Kolehmainen-Aitken, Riitta-Liisa, and Peter Shipp. 1990. "'Indicators of Staffing Need': Assessing Health Staffing and Equity in Papua New Guinea." *Health Policy and Planning* 5 (2): 167–76.

Liu, Xiaoyun, Tim Martineau, Chen Lieping, Zhan Shaokang, Tang Shenglan. 2006. "Does Decentralisation Improve Human Resource Management in the Health Sector? A Case Study from China." *Social Science and Medicine* 63 (7): 1836–45.

Mliga, Gilbert R. 2003. "Decentralization and the Quality of Health Care in Tanzania." In *Africa's Changing Markets for Health and Veterinary Services: The New Institutional Issues*, vol. 5, ed. David K. Leonard. Berkeley: University of California Press. http://repositories.cdlib.org/uciaspubs/editedvolumes/5/8.

Nayyar-Stone, Ritu, Robert Ebel, Sonia Ignatova, and Khalid Rashid, with Harry Hatry and George Peterson. 2006. *Assessing the Impact of Devolution on Healthcare and Education in Pakistan*. Washington, DC: Urban Institute.

Rondinelli, Dennis A., John R. Nellis, and G. Shabbir Cheema. 1984. "Decentralization in Developing Countries: A Review of Recent Experience." World Bank Staff Working Paper 581, World Bank, Washington, DC.

Saltman, Richard B., Vaida Bankauskaite, and Karsten Vrangbaek, eds. 2007. *Decentralization in Health Care: Strategies and Outcomes*. Maidenhead, U.K., and New York: Open University Press.

Simananta, Sima, and Aim-On Aramkul. n.d. "Decentralization of Recruitment in Thai Civil Service." United Nations Public Administration Network, New York. http://unpan1.un.org/intradoc/groups/public/documents/UN/UNPAN 021828.pdf.

Ssengooba, Freddie. 2005. "Human Resources for Health in Decentralized Uganda: Developments and Implications for Health Systems Research." Presentation made at Forum 9, Mumbai, September 12–16.

Steffensen, Jesper, Per Tidemand, Harriet Naitore, Emmanual Ssewankambo, and Eke Mwaipopo. 2004. "Final Synthesis Report: A Comparative Analysis of Decentralisation in Kenya, Tanzania, and Uganda." Working Paper prepared by the Nordic Consulting Group for World Bank, Washington, DC.

Tang, Shenglan, and Gerald Bloom. 2000. "Decentralizing Rural Health Services: A Case Study in China." *International Journal of Health Planning and Management* 15 (3): 189–200.

Thabrany, Hasbullah. 2006. "Human Resources in Decentralized Health Systems in Indonesia: Challenges for Equity." *Regional Health Forum* 10 (1): 75–88.

Turner, Mark M., Owne Podger, Maria S. Sumardjono, and Wayan K. Tirthayasa. 2003. *Decentralisation in Indonesia: Redesigning the State*. Canberra: Asia Pacific Press.

World Bank. 2004. *Health Sector Reform in Bolivia: A Decentralization Case Study*. Washington, DC: World Bank.

World Bank and Asian Development Bank. 2005. *Decentralization in the Philippines: Strengthening Local Government Financing and Resource Management in the Short Term*. Manila: Asian Development Bank.

Review of Alternative Compensation Methods for Health Workers

The global health workforce debate has focused mainly on the shortage of health workers in developing countries and the need to increase staffing. However, mounting evidence indicates that addressing poor health workforce performance—high absenteeism, low productivity, and indifferent quality of care—is an important source of efficiency gains, particularly in the public sector (Hongoro and Normand 2006; Janovsky and Peters 2006; Mathauer and Imhoff 2006). Addressing poor health workforce performance is most important where fiscal constraints may limit the expansion of the health workforce. A key factor that accounts for poor workforce performance in the public sector is the way health workers are paid. Traditionally, health workers in the public sector in developing countries are employed by the national ministry of health and are paid salaries. Salaries are usually based on a national pay scale, and individual salary levels are based primarily on seniority (that is, years of service). Salaries are not tied to any measure of output or performance (Eichler 2006; Hongoro and Normand 2006). Consequently, health workers have very weak incentives to perform at a high level and to achieve the goals of the health system.

This appendix was prepared by Kyla Hayford with inputs from the core team.

Alternative types of payment mechanisms have the potential to provide stronger incentives to health workers and thereby improve performance and efficiency. Developed countries have a long history of alternative payment mechanisms, but only recently have developing countries experimented with innovative compensation policies. This appendix provides a brief overview of the evidence on alternative payment mechanisms for health workers in developing countries and how they affect selected elements of health workforce performance—absenteeism, productivity, and quality of care. It also attempts to lay out the necessary conditions for implementing successful alternative compensation mechanisms to salary. The objective is not to provide a definitive analysis but rather to present some general findings and suggest areas for further work. Although other methods are examined, the focus of this appendix is on performance-based pay.

Rationale for Performance Based Pay

The rationale for why performance-based pay[1] may lead to improved health workforce performance is well established. Health workers respond to incentives. The benefit of performance-based pay is that it aligns the incentives and rewards to health workers with the particular objectives of the district or facility where health workers are employed. The staff is motivated to work toward achieving the goals to obtain the additional compensation when goals are achieved. Theory and evidence show that carefully designed performance-based approaches can align the incentives of the health workers with the societal goals of improving the population's health (Eichler 2006).

Distinguishing performance-based pay and performance-based contracting from contracting out or purchasing of health services is important. Often, performance-based payment for health workers occurs in service delivery units (that is, districts or facilities) that have been contracted by the public sector to provide services. The service delivery units typically have a very high degree of freedom in selecting personnel, hire staff members on a short-term basis, and pay their workers on the basis of performance. Thus, contracting or purchasing health services combines three factors that are likely to significantly affect health workforce performance: the ability to hire and fire staff members, the ability to hire them on a short-term basis, and the ability to pay them on the basis of performance. Therefore, distinguishing the effect of performance-based pay—the focus of this appendix—from the effect of contracting of health services in general is important; they are not the same thing.

Performance-based pay also has several potential drawbacks. It creates the risk of providing unnecessary care because health workers increase their activity to a level that is too high relative to patient needs. This phenomenon is known as *supplier-induced demand*. Indicators on the appropriateness of service are often needed to rein in unnecessary provision. There is also the risk of cost escalation if no measures are put in place. A prevailing weakness of performance indicators is that they often fail to address how well targeted the health care services are. Bonuses are frequently based on improvements in productivity or quality of care, regardless of who receives the services or whether they actually need them (Eichler 2006).

Types of Performance Based Pay

There are several mechanisms through which performance-based pay influences health workforce outcomes. The available evidence focuses on only some of these. Figure D.1 lays out different employment arrangements for health workers that are typical in the public sector. Staff members may be employed directly by the ministry of health or some other national agency. They may be employed by subnational agencies, such as district governments or regional health boards, or they may be directly employed by facilities. In all cases, staff members actually work within a

Figure D.1   Alternative Contracting Arrangements for Health Workers in a Performance-Based Contracting System

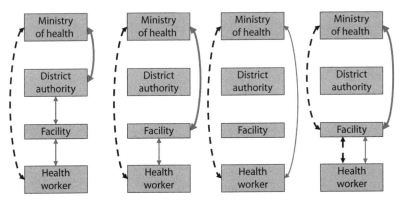

← – → formal employment contract
←→ formal service delivery unit-level performance-based contract
←→ formal or informal individual-level performance-based contract

Source: Author's representation.

facility. The typical compensation method in all cases in the public sector is salary and allowances, few of which are based on performance. Performance-based pay can take several different forms, also illustrated in figure D.1. Staff may directly receive performance-based payments from the ministry of health or relevant national agency. This arrangement means that payment is based directly on individual-level performance. This mechanism is not common in developing countries, but the fee-for-service payment mechanism common in several developed countries is an example. Staff members may also be employed by subnational agencies that have been contracted to provide services, and payments to these agencies are based on the *performance of the agency*. Similarly, the ministry of health or subnational units can contract directly with facilities, and payments to the facility are then based on the *performance of the facility*. Here the situation becomes a bit more complicated. When facilities or subnational units are contracted by the central authority and receive funds on the basis of performance, they often—but not always—have some sort of performance-based payment mechanism for health workers. Many examples of this second model exist in the literature. However, very little information is available on how these facility-level bonuses "trickle down" to health workers and how this remuneration influences individual health worker behavior. In summary, there are few examples in developing countries of direct performance-based pay with the ministry of health or other central authority, many examples of performance-based pay where bonuses are paid to facilities or subnational units, but much less information on how bonus payments are passed on to health workers.

Evidence of the Impact of Performance Based Pay in Practice

In terms of outcomes, the available evidence in the literature focuses on the effect of performance-based pay on health outcomes and health service delivery outcomes. Health workforce outcomes are not examined. The whole impetus behind performance-based pay is to improve health workforce performance (for example, absenteeism, productivity, quality of care), thereby improving service delivery outcomes (for example, immunization rates, skilled birth attendance) and, ultimately, health outcomes of the population (for example, infant mortality). However, the performance-based pay literature has focused mainly on the effect on service delivery and health outcomes and much less on the effect on health workforce performance. This factor is extremely relevant because there is a lack of understanding about how and why some performance-based contracts fail or lead to unintended consequences. Closer examination of health workforce outcomes may help explain this outcome.

The balance of evidence suggests that simply increasing salaries of health workers is not an effective strategy for improving health workforce performance. Salary increases are more effective when tied to performance goals. In low- and middle-income countries, many policy makers assert that extremely low salaries are to blame for high rates of absenteeism, low productivity, and poor quality of care. Although it is true that many health workers are paid well below a living wage, it is not necessarily true that increasing wages will lead to improved performance.[2] Health workers frequently report that low salaries are a barrier to performance, but little evidence shows that increasing their salaries actually brings about better performance (Mathauer and Imhoff 2006). In Malawi, a 52 percent salary top-up for health workers did not have the immediate effect on retention or quality that was expected (Mtonya and Chizimbi 2006). In Ghana, salary increases from the additional duty hours allowance policy failed to reduce health worker emigration (Azeem and Adamtey 2006). Preliminary results from Swaziland, in contrast, suggested that a 60 percent salary increase led to higher retention of public sector doctors and nurses, but the study had no findings on changes in their motivation or performance (Kober and Van Damme 2006). This study suggested that if performance is the goal, the most effective tools will tie financial bonuses to performance outcomes.

Governments can draw from a wide variety of approaches in paying health workers. The options that are feasible will depend on the institutional and legal framework. Other than salary payments, health workers in various countries are paid allowances, fees for service, capitation, performance-based pay, or some mix of methods. As noted earlier, this appendix focuses on the evidence related to performance-based pay. A summary of salary, fee-for-service, and capitation methods is given in box D.1. Governments also need not employ health workers directly at all. They can purchase services from nongovernmental organizations (NGOs) or private providers, as is done in most developed countries. Changing the compensation method for health workers in the public sector may often require legislative reform if the country does not have enough legal and institutional flexibility to be able to reform the civil service system. Romania, Rwanda, and the city of Curitiba, Brazil, have successfully implemented performance-based pay for health workers within the existing public employee system (Vladescu and Radulescu 2001; World Bank 2006). More generally, contracting for health services where health workers are employed by service providers (such as NGOs) and not the government has been successfully implemented in countries as diverse as Cambodia, Guatemala, Haiti, and Uganda (Eichler and others 2007;

Box D.1

Provider Payment Mechanisms and Performance: How Fee-for-Service, Capitation, and Salaried Systems Affect Health Worker Performance

Another way to shape health workers' performance is to redesign the provider payment system in a way that provides incentives for health care providers to behave according to the goals of the health system. Two systematic reviews summarize the important consequences of implementing a fee-for-service (FFS), capitation, or salaried system in developing countries (Gosden, Pedersen, and Torgerson 1999; Gosden and others 2001).

Strong evidence exists that the type of payment mechanism can change incentives and performance of health workers, but the overall health consequences depend on the context and on the way policies were designed. Each type of payment system has its pros and cons. Doctors compensated by FFS tend to be more productive (for example, number of patients seen per month, number of procedures completed per day) and are less likely to be absent than doctors on salary (Gosden, Pedersen, and Torgerson 1999; Gosden and others 2001). Similarly, FFS results in more primary care visits, specialist visits, and curative and diagnostic services but fewer hospital referrals than a capitation system. FFS has better compliance with the recommended number of patient visits than capitation, suggesting that it may improve quality as well as quantity (Gosden and others 2001). A major drawback of FFS is the overprovision of services, which drives up costs for the health system and patients. Capitation typically brings unnecessary care under control, but how capitation or salaried systems affect quality is not clear. Preventive services are more common under salaried or capitation systems than under FFS, suggesting that some quality may be better under these systems (Gosden, Pedersen, and Torgerson 1999).

Depending on the existing problems in a health system, different provider payment approaches can be chosen to shape behavior and address the problem. If underuse is common, FFS may be the best tool for expanding services. If quality of care is a concern, then capitation or salaried systems may be better. In addition to examining how the payment system will affect providers' incentives, governments need to evaluate whether they have the capacity and funding to implement a new system.

Janovsky and Peters 2006; Soeters and Griffiths 2003). In Brazil, for example, the city of Curitiba developed a performance-based scheme within the existing public employee system, whereas the state of São Paulo contracted out to NGOs to deliver health care (World Bank 2006).

Provider groups such as NGOs that are contracted to provide services often have much more flexible hiring arrangements, making the performance-based pay effect difficult to distinguish from the flexible hiring arrangements effect. Health workers in the public sector are typically employed on very secure long-term contracts. This factor often reduces the incentive for good performance because dismissing or sanctioning staff members who perform poorly is difficult. In NGOs, short-term and part-time contracts are used much more extensively. Guyana and Tanzania developed more flexible personnel policies so that retired and part-time workers could reenter the labor force and reduce the burden on existing health workers (Morgan 2005; Rolfe and others 2008). Short-term contracts have also been shown to increase flexibility and accountability of health workers.

The level at which bonuses are paid has an important effect on health worker performance. Individual incentives are the most direct way to promote performance but are the most burdensome to monitor and are therefore less sustainable. Group-based incentives at the facility or subnational level are easier to administer, and they tend to give local managers more autonomy in distributing funds, rewarding individuals, and achieving the performance benchmarks. One drawback of group bonuses is that they can dilute incentives for high performers and reward low-performing free riders, thereby undermining overall performance goals (Hongoro and Normand 2006; Ratto, Propper, and Burgess 2002). To balance the incentive structure, most performance-based pay schemes combine individual and group incentives (Eichler 2006; Soeters and Griffiths 2003).

Performance-based pay at the individual level is the strongest tool for improving performance, but it can be difficult to monitor and sustain. Ministries of health and clinics can pay bonuses to individual health workers for improving their own performance (for example, decreasing absenteeism, meeting attendance patient visits per day goals) or for improving patient health outcomes (for example, immunization coverage, disease incidence). The Democratic Republic of Congo used such bonuses to reward physicians and other health workers. An evaluation of the entire scheme has not been completed, but evidence from one hospital showed a 242 percent increase in medical consultations after performance-based contracts were instituted

(Eichler 2006). Although unnecessary provision of care is a risk, the findings illustrate that performance-based pay to individuals can significantly change providers' behavior. In Cambodia, a more rigorous study found that performance contracts with individual health workers successfully reduced absenteeism and informal payments while improving drug provision and transparency. However, the high costs for the new performance-based payment system strained the hospital budget and undermined the system's sustainability (Soeters and Griffiths 2003).

Incentives need not be monetary. The field of tuberculosis (TB) interventions offers innovative examples of performance-based contracting at the individual level, especially health workers in the private sector. Across many countries, performance-based incentives have improved case management and control of TB (Beith, Eichler, and Weil 2007). An innovative twist on performance-based incentives is the use of nonmonetary incentives or "soft contracts," which exchange goods rather than money for performance. In a review of 15 TB studies that offered publicly provided drugs and training to private providers in exchange for improved TB detection outcomes, 13 of the programs (87 percent) had treatment success rates greater than 80 percent (Lonnroth, Uplekar, and Blanc 2006).

Performance-based pay at the group level—facility or subnational unit—can bring about large and rapid improvements in service delivery outcomes. However, the effect on health workforce performance has not been well documented. When government funding is tied to the performance of a hospital or clinic, improvements in productivity, quality of care, and health outcomes are often observed. A review of 13 studies on contracting NGOs for health care delivery found that seven programs had performance stipulations in the contracts. Two programs offered bonuses for good performance (urban Bangladesh and Haiti) while the other five withdrew bonuses for poor performance (Bolivia, Cambodia, Costa Rica, Madagascar, and Senegal) (Liu, Hotchkiss, and Bose 2008).

Contracting with NGOs for service delivery can achieve better health outcomes at lower costs than making changes in the public sector. Striking examples from urban Bangladesh; Cambodia; Hyderabad, India; and Pakistan found that NGOs achieved better health outcomes when they had the same or fewer resources than public providers (Loevinsohn and Harding 2005).[3] In Bangladesh, areas with NGO service experienced large improvements in quality of care indicators compared with areas served by the public sector (Loevinsohn and Harding

2005). After the introduction of performance-based contracting in Cambodia, the out-of-pocket expenditure on health declined, despite increases in user fees, from US$18 to US$11 per capita. This important finding illustrates that if clinics can provide quality care at a reasonable cost, more households will use public clinics and thus avoid the high costs of unregulated private clinics (Soeters and Griffiths 2003). NGOs might be more successful than the public sector at improving performance and health outcomes for several reasons. NGOs tend to be smaller and more nimble at allocating resources and responding to patient and health system needs. They are less likely to be mired in the procedural or political barriers of the public sector bureaucracy. Also, the competition for contracts between NGOs encourages quality and productivity (Soeters, Habineza, Peerenboom 2006).

The way performance-based payments to facilities affect individual health worker compensation and behavior is not well understood. Despite numerous success stories of performance-based contracting at the level of the service unit, how it affects individual health workers is not well understood. Few studies have illustrated how and if performance bonuses at the hospital or clinic level reach the individual workers. Some exceptions are the cases of Cambodia and Romania, where some information is available (see boxes D.2 and D.3). In Brazil, contracting with NGOs led to improvements in health worker performance and health outcomes, but little or no evidence showed that the superior performance in NGO-run hospitals was due to performance pay or other financial incentives to health workers. Instead, hospital managers believed contracting offered them greater freedom to recruit and hire staff members more appropriately (World Bank 2006). More research is needed on the mechanisms by which bonuses at the facility level lead to changes in performance and motivation of individual health workers.

The effect of performance-based contracting is closely tied to the outcome indicator on which performance is judged. Among the countries that used health workforce performance outcomes as an indicator, clear improvements took place in these outcomes. For example, in urban Bangladesh, contracted NGOs had a higher percentage of clients saying waiting time was acceptable than did public providers (Mahmud, Ullah, and Ahmed 2002). In Haiti, performance contracts with NGOs were associated with a reduction in waiting time for children's health care (Eichler and others 2007). Among the countries that used health outcomes or health service delivery outcomes as indicators of performance, the results

Box D.2

Case Study: Performance Contracts with Physicians in Romania

In the 1990s, the quality of primary care in Romania was improved in part by reforming the physician contracting system. In the old health system, Romanians did not have confidence in public sector primary care services and usually sought care directly from specialists and hospitals. Health care was, in theory, free, but most people made informal payments to receive faster or higher-quality care. Primary care physicians, whose incomes were based on seniority and length of service, had virtually no incentives to provide preventive care or improve patient satisfaction.

As part of a large health sector reform, Romania introduced output-based contracts for primary care physicians in 8 of 40 districts. The scheme aimed to align physicians' incentives with the health sector goals by (a) offering financial incentives to physicians and (b) promoting competition. It sought to strike a balance by specifying an adequate yet monitorable number of performance targets, developing a financially sustainable set of bonuses, and encouraging performance without sacrificing too much flexibility to respond to patients' needs.

To receive a contract, physicians were required to have at least 500 registered patients. This criterion aimed to increase productivity and encourage physicians to move to underserved areas. The ideal number of patients was set at 1,500, and financial incentives were used to encourage physicians not to exceed this threshold. The payment system was a combination of capitation and fee for service. Capitation (60 percent of total payments to physicians) provided an incentive for physicians to keep their patients healthy and to limit unnecessary tests and services. Fee for service (40 percent of payments) encouraged productivity and was used to promote certain procedures (for example, preventive care, immunizations, prenatal care).

In the eight pilot districts, the introduction of output-based contracts resulted in improvements in the number of primary care services offered and in patient satisfaction. Family doctors provided 21 percent more consultations and 40 percent more home visits than before; 87 percent of doctors were providing emergency coverage at night and on weekends. Patients reported that physicians had become more client-oriented and that informal payments had declined. A surprising result was that 80 percent of physicians saw an increase in their salary (average salary increase of 15 percent). But the scheme was not successful in getting physicians to move to underserved areas.

The output-based contracting pilot highlighted three important points. First, the health system needs better monitoring systems. Assessing the quality

(continued)

and monitoring the actual provision of services provided by each doctor were difficult. Second, a stronger regulatory environment is needed to ensure that good performance is rewarded and contract stipulations are enforced. Several districts, for example, awarded contracts to physicians with fewer than 500 patients. Third, recruiting doctors to underserved areas was more difficult than expected. Additional bonuses will be needed if Romania aims to recruit workers to these areas. When Romania scaled up the output-based contracting to the national level, several revisions were made—providing a more detailed yet simplified set of expectations for care under the capitation system, simplifying the fee-for-service payments, offering rewards for effective prevention services (bonus for detecting tuberculosis), increasing discretion over clinic spending, increasing expected patient list to 2,000 individuals, and doubling the capitation payments to doctors who work in remote or low-income areas. Romania's experiment with contracting continues to be revised to meet the evolving needs of the health system.

Source: Vladescu and Radulescu 2001

Box D.3

Case Study: Contracting In and Contracting Out in Cambodia

The Cambodian Basic Health Services Project is one of the most well-designed and well-studied examples of alternative contracting. Before the health reforms in the 1990s, absenteeism, informal payments, dual practice, and drug theft were common, largely because of the extremely poor compensation of health workers. Most salaries were between US$10 and US$12 per month, a mere tenth of the monthly income needed to achieve a basic standard of living (Hongoro and Normand 2006).

In 1996, Cambodia launched the Basic Health Services Project with the dual goals of improving health care access for rural populations and strengthening district-level management. A cornerstone of the approach was to implement performance contracts with NGOs to deliver care. In the pilot study, 12 districts were randomly assigned to one of three types of contracting approaches:

1. *Contracting out.* NGOs were contracted to provide health services and given full control over hiring, firing, and procurement of drugs and supplies.
2. *Contracting in.* NGOs were contracted to manage district-level public facilities but had to work with government staff members and within the government

(continued)

Box D.3 *(Continued)*

procurement system. In addition to publicly provided funds, US$0.25 per capita was provided for staff incentives.

3. *Control group.* No contracting occurred. Traditional management and provision of care were carried out in government facilities by a government staff. Funding was increased by US$0.25 per capita.

After districts were randomized, a competitive bidding process between NGOs was held for districts with contracting-out and contracting-in approaches. Both contract approaches used performance-based incentives to motivate their staff. For example, salaries in one of the contracting-in districts were allocated as follows: 55 percent basic pay, 15 percent punctuality incentive payment, and 30 percent performance bonus (based on achieving monthly financial targets) (Soeters and Griffiths 2003).

Multiple studies found that both the contracting-in and contracting-out models outperformed the control districts. Bhushan and others found that both types of contracting were associated with an increase in prenatal care, delivery in a health facility, and immunization coverage (Bhushan, Keller, and Schwartz 2002). Bloom and others (2006) added that contracting in and contracting out increased the probability that all staff members would be present by 50 and 79 percentage points, respectively. Also, the availability of 24-hour care improved with contracting (Bloom and others 2006). Although the differences between contracting in and contracting out were small, the increased managerial autonomy in the contracting-out model is believed to have accounted for the slightly larger gains in health outcomes.

This Cambodia case study offers rare insight into how clinic-level bonuses trickle down to the health worker. The US$0.25 per capita supplement for the contracting-in NGOs was intended to be used for operating costs, but in reality it was used for staff incentives. The NGOs found motivating the government workers or enforcing regulations difficult without salary bonuses and therefore began offering a fixed bonus as well as a performance-based bonus. The contracting-out NGOs used a different strategy—paying generous fixed salaries (higher than government salaries) without performance bonuses, but using the risk of dismissal as an incentive for performance. Despite very different approaches to hiring and compensating health workers, both contracting approaches achieved similar results. The study also demonstrated that the organizational structure and the design of incentives play a fundamental role in shaping how a contracting system actually unfolds.

Source: Bhushan et al, 2002; Soeters, Robert, and Griffith, 2003.

were mixed. In Madagascar and Senegal, where NGOs were contracted to deliver community-based nutrition services, severe and moderate malnutrition declined by 4 percent and 6 percent, respectively, in the NGO areas (Marek and others 1999). In Haiti, NGOs could receive bonuses up to 10 percent of historical budgets for achieving performance goals. The NGOs with the performance contracts had 13 to 24 percentage point higher immunization coverage and 17 to 27 percentage point higher "attended deliveries" coverage than NGOs without performance stipulations (Eichler and others 2007). However, other studies found mixed or no effect. Performance-based reforms in Costa Rica had no effect on infant mortality rates. In Bangladesh, a rigorous impact evaluation found higher rates of prenatal care and vitamin A and iron supplementation coverage in areas with performance contracts but no difference in nutritional status, weight gain during pregnancy, or birth weight (Garcia-Prado and Chawla 2006; Gauri, Cercone, and Briceño 2005; Operations Evaluation Department 2005). The most rigorous evaluation came from Cambodia, which showed that NGO-run clinics made larger improvements in immunization coverage, prenatal care, and other preventive services than did government-run clinics (Soeters and Griffiths 2003).

More research is needed to show how performance-based bonuses paid to facilities or districts are passed down to health workers. Such research might be an important step in explaining successes and failures. In most studies on performance-based pay, health workforce performance is not measured. Table D.1 illustrates that few studies explicitly evaluate changes in the health workers' performance outcomes—specifically, absenteeism, productivity, and quality of services. Such indicators can be measured more quickly and easily than health outcomes and are more direct tools for evaluating the effect of performance-based contracting. To better explain the mechanism by which contracting approaches affect performance, future studies need to measure health worker outcomes as well as health outputs and outcomes.

Key Messages

The evidence suggests several important conditions that are necessary for performance-based pay to be effective. The effectiveness of performance-based contracts must be evaluated within the political, economic, and institutional context of where they are being implemented (Mills and others 2004). Case studies point to important conditions for implementing a successful program, but no "silver bullets" will ensure that contracting actually results in the intended performance outcomes. Some important

Table D.1 Selected Outcomes Measured in Performance-Based Contracting Interventions

Country	Health workforce outcomes measured	Other health outcomes
Bangladesh (Mahmud, Khan, and Ahmed 2002)	• Percentage of clients reporting that waiting times were acceptable • Percentage of prescriptions provided with a specific diagnosis	• Percentage of health centers providing immunizations • Percentage of health centers providing family planning methods • Percentage of health centers providing hemoglobin lab tests
Cambodia (Soeters and Griffiths 2003)	• Punctuality[a] • Achievement of financial targets[a] • Percentage of correct diagnoses and treatments • Patient perception of quality	• Immunization coverage • Delivery in health facility • Prenatal coverage • Percentage of children with diarrhea receiving oral rehydration salts
Costa Rica (Gauri, Cercone, and Briceño 2005)	• None	• Immunization coverage • Prenatal care coverage • Coverage rates for established interventions for children, elderly, women over 35 years of age
Haiti (Eichler and others 2007)	• Waiting time for patients	• Immunization coverage • Percentage of women using oral rehydration therapy to treat children's diarrhea • Coverage of 3 prenatal visits • Percentage of clinics with more than 3 modern methods of family planning • Percentage of women using oral rehydration therapy correctly • Discontinuation rate for oral and injectable contraceptives

Madagascar (Marek and others 1999)	• Percentage of children weighed monthly	• Percentage of women attending weekly health and nutrition sessions • Percentage of malnourished children • Child anthropometry • Immunization coverage
Romania (Vladescu and Radulescu 2001)	• Patient list of more than 500 people[a] • Number of consultations • Number of household visits	
Rwanda (Soeters, Habineza, and Peerenboom 2006)	• Number of consultations	• Immunization coverage • Prenatal coverage • Contraceptive prevalence rates • Percentage of institutional deliveries
Senegal (Marek and others 1999)	• Percentage of children weighed monthly	• Percentage of women attending weekly health and nutrition sessions • Percentage of malnourished children • Child anthropometry

Sources: Authors' compilation based on sources listed.

a. The outcome was specified in a performance-based contract. Achievement of these outcomes was used to determine performance-based compensation for the health worker or for the clinic or hospital. For some countries, outcomes used for granting performance bonuses were not specified.

lessons learned from previous experiments with performance-based contracting include the following:

- *A supportive legal framework and government flexibility are required.* For many low- and middle-income countries, performance-based policies fail because of political, legal, and institutional barriers to such reforms. Reducing or reorganizing the civil service may be politically too difficult (Hongoro and Normand 2006). Governments may also have their hands tied by restrictive laws on hiring and compensating civil servants. In São Paulo, Brazil, hospital managers argued that their success with contracting was largely due to the autonomy they had in hiring, promoting, and firing their employees (World Bank 2006). Without such flexibility or an enabling legal environment, the options for alternative contracting will be limited.

- *Adequate management skills are needed at all levels.* In fragile states or countries with weak governance, the "contract and incentivize" approach is recommended over the "command and control" approach because the former requires less institutional capacity at the federal level (Eichler 2006). Yet it should be underscored that performance-based contracting cannot be implemented in the absence of adequate management skills—especially at the district and local levels. Hospitals and clinics need to have sufficient management capacity to motivate and evaluate their employees. The ministries of health also need sufficient capacity to oversee and administer the often complicated contracts. For contracting out to NGOs, a strong NGO sector with technical and managerial skills must exist in the country (Eichler 2006). Performance-based incentives require accountability and credible enforcement. Without them, contracting could inadvertently lead to increased inefficiency, decreased transparency, and corruption.

- *Adequate monitoring capacity is needed.* When contracts are linked to performance, monitoring must be frequent and effective (Soeters and Griffiths 2003). Performance-based contracts—especially those implemented at the individual level—require nontrivial levels of commitment and skill for monitoring and evaluation. Many health systems do not have the databases, measurement tools, or human capital in place to do ongoing surveillance of individual health workers' performance. For low-skill or resource-constrained settings, contracting at the service unit level may be more feasible.

- *Appropriately targeted incentives are needed.* One of the largest challenges of developing a performance-based contracting scheme is designing incentives that will lead to the socially desirable and intended performance outcomes. A pilot program in Cambodia revealed that its performance-based incentives for individuals were set too low to affect staff behavior significantly (Soeters and Griffiths 2003). In Romania, incentives to encourage doctors to work in rural areas failed because they were too small and inappropriately targeted (Vladescu and Radulescu 2001). Also, poorly planned incentives can lead to socially undesirable outcomes. In China, performance bonuses to doctors appeared to increase the provision of unnecessary services and drugs and, in some cases, to reduce productivity (Liu and Mills 2005). Reforms to improve management in Costa Rica actually led to an increase in absenteeism, in part because of unintended consequences of tweaking the incentive structure (Garcia-Prado and Chawla 2006). Thus, designing a performance-based approach requires great care in examining the potentially beneficial and perverse consequences. Although the focus of this appendix is the health worker, the effects on other stakeholders and other aspects of care (for example, equity and access) should also be taken into account (Liu, Hotchkiss, and Bose 2008).

In summary, the balance of evidence shows that pay for performance at both the individual and facility levels could be a very effective way of improving health workforce performance in the public sector. When compensation of health workers is tied to performance, significant improvements in health workforce performance and service delivery outcomes can occur. However, performance-based pay requires careful selection of indicators that performance will be measured against and careful design of incentives so that they align health worker behavior with the goals of the health system. Many countries have experimented with performance-based pay, and it is clear that monitoring capacity, management capacity, and a flexible institutional and legal framework are important factors for success.

Notes

1. *Performance-based pay* is defined as any payment that is "conditional on taking a measurable action or achieving a predetermined performance target" (Eichler 2006: 5).

2. Before Cambodia's New Deal reforms in 2000, public sector health workers earned one-tenth of what is considered the minimum salary needed to maintain basic living standards.

3. Not all these examples have explicit performance stipulations in the contracts.

References

Azeem, Vitus, and Nicholas Adamtey. 2006. *Budget Ceilings and Health in Ghana.* Amsterdam: Integrated Social Development Centre.

Beith, Alexandra, Rena Eichler, and Diana Weil. 2007. "Performance-Based Incentives for Health: A Way to Improve Tuberculosis Detection and Treatment Completion?" Working Paper 122, Center for Global Development, Washington, DC.

Bhushan, Indu, Sheryl Keller, and Brad Schwartz. 2002. "Achieving the Twin Objectives of Efficiency and Equity: Contracting Health Services in Cambodia." Economics and Research Department Brief 6, Asian Development Bank, Manila.

Bloom, Erik, Indu Bhushan, David Clingingsmith, Rathavuth Hong, Elizabeth King, Michael Kremer, Benjamin Loevinsohn, and J. Brad Schwartz. 2006. *Contracting for Health: Evidence from Cambodia.* Washington, DC: Brookings Institution.

Eichler, Rena. 2006. "Can 'Pay for Performance' Increase Utilization by the Poor and Improve the Quality of Health Services?" Discussion paper for the first meeting of the Working Group on Performance-Based Incentives, Center for Global Development, Washington, DC, February 7.

Eichler, Rena, Paul Auxila, Uder Antoine, and Bernateau Desmangles. 2007. "Performance-Based Incentives for Health: Six Years of Results from Supply-Side Programs in Haiti." Working Paper 121, Center for Global Development, Washington, DC.

Garcia-Prado, Ariadna, and Mukesh Chawla. 2006. "The Impact of Hospital Management Reforms on Absenteeism in Costa Rica." *Health Policy and Planning* 21 (2): 91–100.

Gauri, Varun, James Cercone, and Rodrigo Briceño. 2005. "Contracting Primary Health Care Services: The Case of Costa Rica." In *Health Systems Innovation in Central America: Lessons and Impact of New Approaches,* ed. Gerry La Forgia. Washington, DC: World Bank.

Gosden, Toby, Frode Forland, Ivar Sonbo Kristiansen, Matthew Sutton, Brenda Leese, Antonio Giuffrida, Michelle Sergison, and Lone Pedersen. 2001. "Impact of Payment Method on Behaviour of Primary Care Physicians: A Systematic Review." *Journal of Health Services Research and Policy* 6 (1): 44–55.

Gosden, Toby, Lone Pedersen, and David Torgerson. 1999. "How Should We Pay Doctors? A Systematic Review of Salary Payments and Their Effect on Doctor Behaviour." *QJM: Monthly Journal of the Association of Physicians* 92 (1): 47–55.

Hongoro, Charles, and Charles Normand. 2006. "Health Workers: Building and Motivating the Workforce." In *Disease Control Priorities in Developing Countries*, ed. Dean T. Jamison, Joel G. Breman, Anthony R. Measham, George Alleyne, Mariam Claeson, David B. Evans, Prabhat Jha, Anne Mills, and Philip Musgrove, 1309–22. New York: Oxford University Press.

Janovsky, Katja, and David Peters. 2006. "Improving Health Services and Strengthening Health Systems: Adopting and Implementing Innovative Strategies." Working Paper 5, Department of Health Policy, Development and Services Evidence and Information for Policy, World Health Organization, Geneva.

Kober, Katharina, and Wim Van Damme. 2006. "Public Sector Nurses in Swaziland: Can the Downturn Be Reversed?" *Human Resources for Health* 4: 13.

Liu, Xingzhu, David R. Hotchkiss, and Sujata Bose. 2008. "The Effectiveness of Contracting Out Primary Health Care Services in Developing Countries: A Review of the Evidence." *Health Policy and Planning* 23 (1): 1–13.

Liu, Xingzhu, and Anne Mills. 2005. "The Effect of Performance-Related Pay of Hospital Doctors on Hospital Behaviour: A Case Study from Shandong, China." *Human Resources for Health* 3: 11.

Loevinsohn, Benjamin, and April Harding. 2005. "Buying Results? Contracting for Health Service Delivery in Developing Countries." *Lancet* 366 (9486): 676–81.

Lonnroth, Knut, Mukund Uplekar, and Leopold Blanc. 2006. "Hard Gains through Soft Contracts: Productive Engagement of Private Providers in Tuberculosis Control." *Bulletin of the World Health Organization* 84 (11): 876–83.

Mahmud, Hasib, Amanat Ullah Khan, and Salahuddin Ahmed. 2002. *Mid-Term Health Facility Survey: Urban Primary Health Care Project*. Dhaka: Mitra and Associates.

Marek, Tonia, Issakha Diallo, Biram Ndiaye, and Jean Rakotosalama. 1999. "Successful Contracting of Prevention Services: Fighting Malnutrition in Senegal and Madagascar." *Health Policy and Planning* 14 (4): 382–89.

Mathauer, Inke, and Ingo Imhoff. 2006. "Health Worker Motivation in Africa: The Role of Non-financial Incentives and Human Resource Management Tools." *Human Resources for Health* 4: 24.

Mills, Anne, Natasha Palmer, Lucy Gilson, Di McIntyre, Helen Schneider, Edina Sinanovic, and Haroon Wadee. 2004. "The Performance of Different Models of Primary Care Provision in Southern Africa." *Social Science and Medicine* 59 (5): 931–43.

Morgan, Rachael. 2005. "Addressing Health Worker Shortages: Recruiting Retired Nurses to Reduce Mother-to-Child Transmission in Guyana." Family Health International, Institute for HIV/AIDS, Arlington, VA.

Mtonya, Brian, and Steven Chizimbi. 2006. *Systemwide Effects of the Global Fund in Malawi: Final Report.* Bethesda, MD: Partners for Health Reform*plus* Project, Abt Associates.

Operations Evaluation Department. 2005. Maintaining Momentum to 2015? An Impact Evaluation of Interventions to Improve Maternal and Child Health and Nutrition Outcomes in Bangladesh. Washington, DC: World Bank.

Ratto, Marisa, Carol Propper, and Simon Burgess. 2002. "Using Financial Incentives to Promote Teamwork in Health Care." *Journal of Health Services Research and Policy* 7 (2): 69–70.

Rolfe, Ben, Sebalda Leshabari, Fredrik Rutta, and Susan F. Murray. 2008. "The Crisis in Human Resources for Health Care and the Potential of a 'Retired' Workforce: Case Study of the Independent Midwifery Sector in Tanzania." *Health Policy and Planning* 23 (2): 137–49.

Soeters, Robert, and Fred Griffiths. 2003. "Improving Government Health Services through Contract Management: A Case from Cambodia." *Health Policy and Planning* 18 (1): 74–83.

Soeters, Robert, Christian Habineza, and Peter Bob Peerenboom. 2006. "Performance-Based Financing and Changing the District Health System: Experience from Rwanda." *Bulletin of the World Health Organization* 84 (11): 884–89.

Vladescu, Cristian, and Silviu Radulescu. 2001. "Improving Primary Health Care: Output-Based Contracting in Romania." Viewpoint, World Bank, Washington, DC.

World Bank. 2006. *Brazil: Enhancing Performance in Brazil's Health Sector— Lessons from Innovations in the State of São Paulo and the City of Curitiba.* Washington, DC: World Bank.

Review of GFATM Round 6 and GAVI HSS Round 1 Policies and Practices for Funding Health Worker Remuneration

In recent years, the international community has committed to scaling up aid for health. Development assistance for health has risen steadily since 1990 from about US$2 billion to more than US$10 billion in 2003. Much of the post-2000 increase can be credited to an increasing number of global partnerships and a significant rise in private philanthropic funding. Partnerships and philanthropies have joined efforts to increase awareness and financing aimed at the eradication of major diseases. Global programs such as the Global Fund to Fight AIDS, Tuberculosis, and Malaria (GFATM); the Global Alliance for Vaccines and Immunization (GAVI); Roll Back Malaria; and the U.S. President's Emergency Plan for AIDS Relief (PEPFAR), as well as several others, represented roughly 15 percent of total health aid in 2002 and 20 percent in 2003 (Gottret and Schieber 2006). In theory, the large inflows of donor assistance for health could be used as an additional source of financing for the health wage bill, creating more fiscal space for hiring health workers.

In the area of human resources for health (HRH), donor assistance has traditionally focused on training activities rather than on funding

This appendix was prepared by Sherry Madan with inputs from the core team.

additional hiring (that is, salaries of health workers). For example, a review of GFATM grants found that, in general, most countries do not sufficiently use the possibilities that the GFATM provides for health system strengthening and human resource interventions, even though a great majority of proposals recognize improving human resource constraints as key to the success of future interventions. Most proposals include some activities to address human resource constraints. The most frequent activity is training, focused mainly on short-term, in-service training. Support for preservice training and training institutions is rare, and hardly any long-term strategies are proposed to address the lack of adequately trained personnel. Recruitment plans are also frequently included, but in most cases they are limited to a small number of staff members at the program management level and do not address the shortages at the service delivery level (Dräger, Gedik, and Dal Poz 2006).

This appendix examines the policies and practices of two major donor agencies in the health sector: GFATM and GAVI. The following key questions are explored:

- What are the policies of each of the agencies regarding funding of health worker remuneration (that is, salaries, allowances, and per diems)?
- To what extent are countries using these two sources of financing to fund remuneration of health workers?
- What are some of the labor market implications associated with these practices?

The guidelines for funding applications for GFATM and GAVI Health Systems Strengthening (HSS) were reviewed. All GFATM Round 6 grant applications[1] and all GAVI HSS Round 1 approved grants were reviewed for their HRH content. Finally, the reports of the grant review committees in each agency were reviewed to identify the quality of the HRH activities in the proposals and whether they were consistent with those outlined in the guidelines. This work builds on that of Dräger, Gedik, and Dal Poz (2006), who were the first to examine human resource content in GFATM grants in a sample of African countries. The analysis extends their work by examining all GFATM Round 6 applications and GAVI HSS grants as well. The type of remuneration is also examined in much more detail (that is, salary payments for new positions that are fully funded, per diems, and salary top-ups for existing health workers) as are sustainability issues. Finally, the available evidence on the labor market effects is reviewed.

GFATM and GAVI Policies on Remuneration

GFATM and GAVI—the two agencies examined—have quite flexible policies toward funding health worker remuneration. However, a key condition is sustainability. Both agencies have increasingly recognized the importance of addressing health workforce issues to achieve results. The GFATM guidelines for Round 7 proposals say that HRH activities will be funded if a strong link between the proposed activities and health systems strengthening as well as the three target diseases can be demonstrated (GFATM 2007). It is also essential that the proposal outline the sustainability of the activities at the end of the proposal period. The guidelines clearly indicate remuneration is eligible but state that in cases where human resources are an important share of the budget, the proposal must explain (a) to what extent such spending will strengthen health systems' capacity at the patient or target population level and (b) how the salaries will be sustained after the proposal period is over (GFATM 2007).

In the proposals, GFATM requires that the proposed intervention be linked to long-term HRH development. GFATM also expects a clear human resource development plan, identification of gaps, a link between human resources and target disease coverage, a needs assessment, and integration with disease-specific national plans.

The GAVI guidelines highlight "health workforce mobilization, distribution and motivation targeted at those engaged in immunization, and other health services at the district level and below" (GAVI Alliance 2007: 5) as one of three major priority areas for funding. The guidelines state that "GAVI HSS support can be used for one-off expenditures that increase system capacity" (GAVI Alliance 2007: 7), such as pay for performance, contracting with nongovernmental organizations (NGOs), and training and technical support, as well as for recurrent expenditures such as fuel, maintenance, and per diems for outreach. Sustainability of these expenditures when GAVI HSS funds are no longer available must be demonstrated.

To get a sense of the extent to which countries are using GAVI HSS and GFATM grants to pay health workers, this research reviewed Round 1 GAVI HSS approved grants and Round 6 GFATM applications. The methods of remuneration were also reviewed.

Country Practices

The share of GAVI HSS and GFATM funding used for payments to staff members varies widely across countries. On average, countries devote 12 percent of GAVI HSS and 16 percent of GFATM funds for paying health workers. However, this amount ranges from 0 to 28 percent (Kenya) within GAVI HSS and from 0 to 46 percent (Indonesia for malaria) within GFATM. Within GFATM, the share devoted to payments to staff members is quite consistent over the different disease priorities. Within GAVI HSS, part of the variation is because the size of the HRH component varies widely, and within the HRH component, the focus also varies (that is, among training, payments to staff members, and other activities). Clearly, some countries are quite aggressively using GAVI HSS funds for payments to health workers. In Burundi, the entire GAVI HSS grant is being used to pay staff members.

The method of remuneration for payments to staff members within GAVI HSS and GFATM grants is diverse. The most common form of remuneration within GFATM grants is salary payments. In only 20 percent of grants does one find any payment of allowances and per diems or performance-based incentives (figure E.1).[2] Within GAVI HSS, allowances and performance-based incentives are used much more extensively. For example, 100 percent of the Burundi grant is used for payments to staff members, and the entire amount is used to pay performance-based incentives to health workers. Salary payments are much less common (figure E.2).

A significant portion of payments to staff members in both GAVI HSS and GFATM grants are for frontline health workers. However, remuneration methods for these frontline health workers are different and suggest differences in the effect on the health workforce. More than 30 percent of GFATM grants have some share of their budget devoted to paying frontline health workers, and 36 percent pay administrative and managerial staff members. Five of the six GAVI HSS grants supported payments to frontline health workers. However, within GAVI, the remuneration payments to frontline health workers are mostly in the form of allowances, sometimes performance-based. Within GFATM, however, most of the remuneration to frontline health workers is in the form of salaries (figure E.3). This analysis suggests that GAVI HSS grants focus more on supplementing the income and improving the performance of the current health workforce, whereas the GFATM grants focus more on creating newly funded positions, thereby expanding the health workforce.

Depending on the aid modality, wage distortions can occur, resulting in unintended consequences regarding staffing. But good coordination can mitigate this outcome. When funding agencies pay salaries and allowances to health workers, such action can create large wage differences between

Figure E.1   Share of GFATM (Round 6) Grants Used for Remuneration of Health Workers

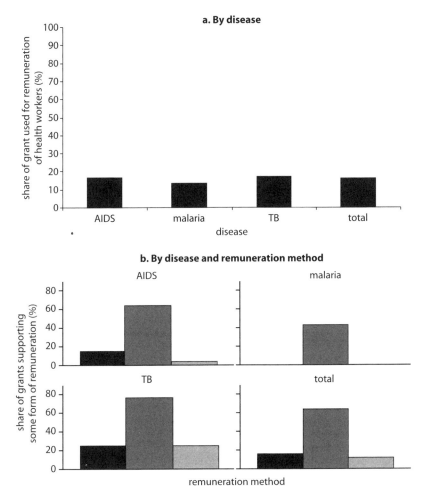

Source: Authors' analysis of GFATM Round 6 applications.

programs that are funded through external support and those that are not. Whether this outcome occurs depends crucially on whether funds are channeled through the government or, if they are not, on how closely the external funding agencies coordinate with the government. For example, if agencies agree to provide similar pay and benefits to health

Figure E.2   Share of GAVI HSS (Round 1) Grants Used for Remuneration of Health Workers

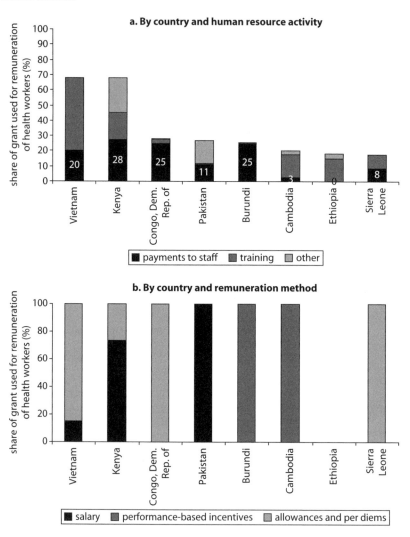

Source: Authors' analysis of GFATM Round 6 applications.

workers as those in the public sector, then wage distortions will be minimized. In fact, both GAVI HSS and GFATM, which are both highly coordinated with the government, are well positioned to avoid these distortions. Agencies such as PEPFAR, which primarily funds NGOs, are more likely to promote wage distortions. Recent experience in Kenya

Figure E.3   Method of Payments to Managerial and Frontline Staff Members within GFATM (Round 6) Grants

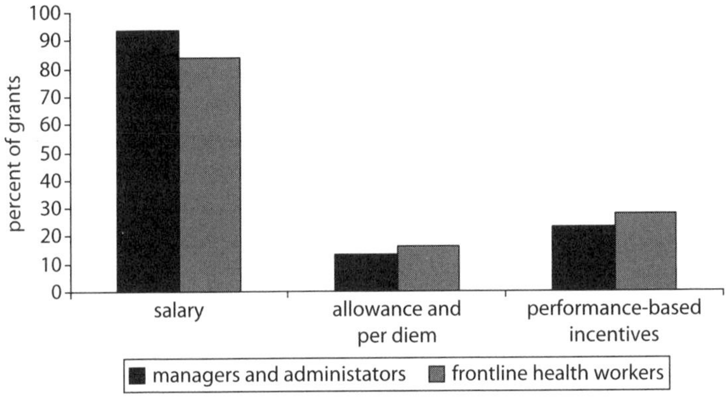

Source: Authors' analysis of GFATM Round 6 applications.

shows that when donors support hiring through pooled funds, use existing pay scales within the public sector, and agree not to recruit staff from certain agencies, the negative wage distortions are avoided (box E.1).

Some emerging evidence indicates wage distortions in some countries. However, further work is needed in this area. In Ethiopia, for example, a review of the GFATM experience suggested that jobs in HIV-related services became more attractive after GFATM resources became available (Banteyerga, Kidanu, and Stillman 2006). In Benin, evidence indicates that facilities supported through GFATM grants followed the government pay scale and had just as much trouble attracting staff as government facilities. Very little labor movement out of government facilities occurred (Smith and others 2005). A recent analysis of wages in several countries found that government salaries did not match those in the donor and nongovernmental sectors. For example, a driver for a bilateral agency in Addis Ababa was paid more than a professor in the medical faculty, and a government public health specialist could earn four to five times more by joining an international nongovernmental organization (McCoy and others 2008).

Key Considerations in Using GFATM and GAVI Funds for Remuneration

Donor funding of salaries can create contingent liabilities for the government's budget. If donor funds flow through the government budget and are used to hire health workers on permanent contracts, then when the

Box E.1

Examples of Countries Using GFATM Grants to Pay Health Workers

Ukraine AIDS

Human resource costs represent 38 percent of the overall grant budget. These costs mainly support salaries and incentives for multidisciplinary teams performing prevention outreach (social workers, coordinators, psychologists, physicians, and nurses); for antiretroviral therapy and sexually transmitted infection programs (physicians and specialists); and for care and support programs (narcologists, infectionists, physicians, nurses, social workers, and counselors). The proposal will also engage personnel for overall project management (project directors, accountants, and office managers) and for local coordination and capacity building (municipal HIV/AIDS coordinators). The majority of these personnel will be engaged through NGOs, which will be responsible for fund-raising or securing funding from local governments for continuation of activities beyond the grant period.

China AIDS

Human resource costs represent 36 percent of the overall grant budget. These funds are mainly for paying health workers doing outreach, peer education, and counseling within grassroots NGOs. The grant has identified that sustainability for NGO projects and staff members is difficult to resolve. (No information is provided on how this issue will be addressed.)

Vietnam AIDS

Human resource costs represent 18 percent of the overall grant budget. Incentives to supplement government salaries will be provided for 202 staff members at the provincial level, 781 staff members at the district level, 784 mass organization volunteers and health care collaborators at the commune level, and 468 people living with HIV/AIDS collaborators. In addition, the grant will cover salary costs for 15 staff members working in the project management unit. (No indication is made whether the salary supplements will continue after the grant expires.)

Kenya TB

Human resource costs represent 28 percent of the overall grant budget. Most of the resources will be used to hire lab technologists, nurses, and clinical officers to strengthen diagnosis and treatment of tuberculosis (TB) patients at the peripheral health facilities. Though the amount request to pay the staff is for five years only, the government of Kenya is expected to absorb these health workers after Round 6 funding runs out.

India TB

Human resource costs represent 27 percent of the overall grant budget. Additional human resources in the states are limited and cannot adequately undertake supervision, monitoring, and quality assurance activities. The program strengthens the states' capacity by funding recruitment of technical supervisory staff members on a contractual basis at the state, district, and subdistrict levels.

Lesotho TB

Human resource costs represent 25 percent of the overall grant budget. Resources will be used to develop a human resource development plan, including preventive measures to decrease staff turnover. Teams will be recruited to carry out activities at the district level as part of district health teams. Staff members will be paid monthly salaries, and the Ministry of Health will absorb the salaries after five years.

Source: Authors' analysis of GFATM Round 6 applications.

donor funding expires, the government will assume a financial obligation for remuneration payments. If, however, health workers are hired on short-term contracts, the government has more flexibility in adjusting staffing levels in response to donor aid flows because donor aid for health is volatile, unpredictable, and short term (for example, GFATM grants are for a period of at most five years). Short-term contracts are not extensively used in the public sector. Thus, the current donor aid architecture and the contracting arrangements within the public sector pose a challenge in not creating contingent liabilities for the government.

Some emerging practices are promising. In Kenya, resources from several donors were pooled and used to expand hiring of health workers through the Emergency Hiring Program. Health workers were recruited and paid according to the government pay scale, but they were hired on three-year contracts to match the term of the donor support. In Malawi, an initiative led by the U.K. Department for International Development provided significant resources to the government to increase salaries of health workers.

The resources were provided through direct budget support and for a period of six years—much longer than traditional commitments.

Within GFATM and GAVI HSS, sustainability issues surrounding payment of salaries and allowances to frontline health workers are not adequately addressed. Sustainability issues can be dealt with in several ways. Health workers who are paid salaries can be hired on short-term contracts. Allowances can be paid only during the time of the grants. The government can also commit to take over payment of salaries of newly hired staff members or pay allowances after grant funding runs out. The analysis of Round 6 applications shows that when GFATM resources are used to pay either salary or allowances to frontline health workers, in 56 percent of cases there is an assumption that the government will absorb the salary and allowance payments at the end of the grant period, but the government makes no explicit agreement to do so.[3] In no cases has the government made a formal pledge to set aside the necessary budget resources, and in only 9 percent of cases are short-term contracts matching the term of the grant used exclusively. Within GAVI, the issue of sustainability is not dealt with adequately either (Health System Strengthening Independent Review Committee 2007).

Sustainability, the likely success of the intervention, and links to an overall national HRH strategy are some of the main reasons more GAVI and GFATM funding is not used to pay health workers. Within GAVI HSS proposals, one of the main issues identified was the sustainability of staff incomes—either in the cases where staff members will be hired into a separate project management unit or where incomes of frontline health workers are being topped up in various ways (Health System Strengthening Independent Review Committee 2007). The report of the Technical Review Panel for Round 6 of GFATM found that the overall quality of the HRH interventions is poor (GFATM 2006). The panel did not see that they were based on a clear government strategy for overall human resources for health. Sustainability is very important. Funds are for three to five years, but whether the hiring is short term or long term is not clear. The panel suggested the following points be taken into account in guiding future proposals for the funding of remuneration: proposals for salary support and premiums within the public sector and NGOs (a) should take into account the overall human resource policy of the relevant institutions, (b) should use existing salary scales, (c) should minimize negative impact on other aspects of the health care system, and (d) should plan to shift the salary costs to the national budget and provide a clear timetable for doing so. There is also a need to better demonstrate clear benefits to treatment of diseases of GFATM and for immunization in case of GAVI.

Notes

1. At the time the data were collected, it was not possible to know which applications had been approved. The analysis did not look into differences in human resources for health content between approved and rejected applications in both GFATM and GAVI HSS.

2. The breakdown of the budget by salary, per diem, allowances, and the like is not available in GFATM applications, but by reviewing the description of activities funded, one can determine whether salaries, allowances, or performance-based incentives are paid.

3. Given the emphasis on sustainability in the GFATM guidelines, this figure is likely to be much higher among approved applications. All applications were examined for the analysis in this report.

References

Banteyerga, Hailom, Aklilu Kidanu, and Kate Stillman. 2006. *The Systemwide Effects of the Global Fund in Ethiopia: Final Study Report.* Bethesda, MD: Partners for Health Reform*plus* Project, Abt Associates.

Dräger, Sigrid, Gulin Gedik, and Mario R. Dal Poz. 2006. "Health Workforce Issues and the Global Fund to Fight Aids, Tuberculosis, and Malaria: An Analytical Review." *Human Resources for Health* 4: 23. http://www.human-resources-health.com/content/4/1/23.

GAVI Alliance. 2007. "Revised Guidelines for: GAVI Alliance Health System Strengthening (HSS) Applications." GAVI Alliance, Geneva. http://www.gavialliance.org/resources/HSS_Guidelines_2007.pdf.

GFATM (Global Fund to Fight Aids, Tuberculosis and Malaria). 2006. "Report of the Technical Review Panel and the Secretariat on Round 6 Proposals." 14th Board Meeting, Guatemala City, October 31–November 3.

———. 2007. "Guidelines for Proposals Round 7." GFATM, Geneva.

Gottret, Pablo, and George Schieber. 2006. *Health Financing Revisited: A Practitioner's Guide.* Washington, DC: World Bank.

Health System Strengthening Independent Review Committee. 2007. "Report of the Health System Strengthening Independent Review Committee to the Executive Committee." GAVI, Independent Review Committee for HSS, Geneva.

McCoy, David, Sara Bennett, Sophie Witter, Bob Pond, Brook Baker, Jeff Gow, Sudeep Chand, Tim Ensor, and Barbara McPake. 2008. "Salaries and Incomes of Health Workers in Sub-Saharan Africa." *Lancet* 371 (9613): 675–81.

Smith, Owen, Sourou Gbangbade, Assomption Hounsa, and Lynne Miller-Franco. 2005. Bénin: Les Impacts du Fonds Mondial Sur le Système de Santé—Résultats Préliminaires. Bethesda, MD: Partners for Health Reform*plus* Project, Abt Associates.

Index

Boxes, figures, notes, and tables are denoted by b, f, n, and t, following the page numbers.

265

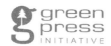